ENDORSEMENT

"Mariza Ferreira and Rebecca Howell have provided a masterclass in inclusive practice for occupational therapists. Their holistic DME-C approach is endorsed by families for its life-changing impact, particularly for children with 'spiky profiles' where it can be difficult to determine the most effective therapeutic interventions. Radiating the spirit of occupational therapy, this book moves beyond labels to focus on practical solutions, such as the 10 Golden Nuggets, helping therapists to identify and support children with DME as a routine part of their professional practice. This book is a must-read for every occupational therapist."

– **Professor Adam Boddison OBE**, co-author of *The School Handbook for DME*

"An essential handbook for occupational therapists working with or interested in working with children who demonstrate characteristics of DME/2e! Written collaboratively by expert DME/2e practitioners, this comprehensive book guides the therapist through clearly structured chapters with detailed information on the identification of DME/2e with easy to use checklists, and tried and tested intervention techniques. Utilising the 10 Golden Nuggets with the 4 Essential Components of the DME-C therapy approach provides the therapist with skills to deliver holistic therapy that embraces the child as an equal partner in the process. I wish this book had been published before I retired!"

– **Sue Davis,** retired independent paediatric occupational therapist

"This is a breakthrough book which offers a practical framework and simple steps to both identify dual and multiple exceptionality and to supplement current professional OT practice to address appropriately the specific issues these children and young people face. Not only that, but I believe that every professional across the practice spectrum, parent/carer and teacher should be aware of the approach outlined in this book. Used in the right way, it could have a major impact on issues ranging from school phobia to behavioural issues at home or in the classroom; mental health challenges to issues related to underachievement and beyond."

– **Denise Yates,** author of *Parenting Dual Exceptional Children* and co-author of *The School Handbook for Dual and Multiple Exceptionali'*

Occupational Therapy for Children with DME or Twice Exceptionality is accompanied by a number of printable online materials designed to ensure this resource best supports your professional needs.

Go to https://resourcecentre.routledge.com/speechmark and click on the cover of this book.

Answer the question prompt using your copy of the book to gain access to the online content.

OCCUPATIONAL THERAPY FOR CHILDREN WITH DME OR TWICE EXCEPTIONALITY

Children with high learning potential or giftedness have remarkable potential. Despite this, these children can struggle to participate in everyday life because of a range of needs that are sometimes misunderstood, overlooked or not adequately addressed, leading to underachievement and, in turn, low self-esteem. Needs that, in many cases, paediatric occupational therapists are best suited to address.

The practical resource offered in the book, the DME-C approach, is a tried-and-tested approach to help children who have challenges relating to their high learning potential, as well as sensory processing differences, unhelpful thought patterns and self-regulation. It draws on the heart of occupational therapy that considers the whole profile of the child, actively caters to the unique profiles of children with dual or multiple exceptionality (DME) or twice exceptionality (2e), and guides therapists towards therapy provision that is strengths-based and achieves favourable outcomes. This book:

- Includes a clear and comprehensive introduction to high learning potential and DME or twice exceptionality (2e), along with guidance to help identify children with these profiles.
- Covers questions and concerns occupational therapists may have when working with children with DME or 2e.
- Considers the similarities and differences between high learning potential/DME/2e and neurodivergent conditions such as developmental coordination disorder, autism and ADHD, with a focus on sensory processing differences.
- Explains, in easy-to-understand language, the full DME-C therapy approach, with a range of example activities to use in therapy to achieve its principles, and a suggested therapy progression plan.
- Is packed full of real-life case studies to translate theory into practice.
- Empowers therapists and educational professionals further by drawing attention to how they can better relate to children with DME/2e in therapy regardless of the children's specific needs.

Full of examples and with the voices of parents and children at its heart, this resource is essential reading for occupational therapists, SENCOs, education psychologists and other relevant professionals who want to improve the lives and wellbeing of children with DME or twice exceptionality and help them reach their full potential.

Mariza Ferreira is passionate about supporting children with DME/2e to reach their full potential. It has become her professional mission to both advocate for these children and highlight the importance of the occupational therapy profession to help them. Mariza provides treatment for children and trains parents and other professionals on child-related topics. She also provides supervision to other occupational therapists. Her motto is to change the world one child at a time. This book is one of the ways she is doing that.

Rebecca Howell is a consultant in educational leadership specialising in governance, policy, risk and systems. Formerly Director of the DME Trust and senior education consultant at Potential Plus UK, she has supported many children with high learning potential and dual and multiple exceptionality and their families. Rebecca is dedicated to driving system-wide improvement in education through collaborative, values-led leadership.

OCCUPATIONAL THERAPY FOR CHILDREN WITH DME OR TWICE EXCEPTIONALITY

A Practical Approach to Support High Learning Potential, Sensory Processing Differences and Self-Regulation

Mariza Ferreira and Rebecca Howell

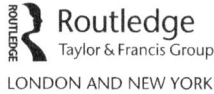

LONDON AND NEW YORK

Designed cover image and all illustrations: Lani Jacobs

First published 2024
by Routledge
4 Park Square, Milton Park, Abingdon, Oxon OX14 4RN

and by Routledge
605 Third Avenue, New York, NY 10158

Routledge is an imprint of the Taylor & Francis Group, an informa business

© 2024 Mariza Ferreira and Rebecca Howell

The right of Mariza Ferreira and Rebecca Howell to be identified as authors of this work has been asserted in accordance with sections 77 and 78 of the Copyright, Designs and Patents Act 1988.

All rights reserved. The purchase of this copyright material confers the right on the purchasing institution to photocopy or download pages which bear the support material icon and a copyright line at the bottom of the page. No other parts of this book may be reprinted or reproduced or utilised in any form or by any electronic, mechanical, or other means, now known or hereafter invented, including photocopying and recording, or in any information storage or retrieval system, without permission in writing from the publishers.

Trademark notice: Product or corporate names may be trademarks or registered trademarks, and are used only for identification and explanation without intent to infringe.

British Library Cataloguing-in-Publication Data
A catalogue record for this book is available from the British Library

ISBN: 978-1-032-36619-7 (hbk)
ISBN: 978-1-032-36616-6 (pbk)
ISBN: 978-1-003-33403-3 (ebk)

DOI: 10.4324/9781003334033

Typeset in Interstate
by Deanta Global Publishing Services, Chennai, India

Access the Support Material: https://resourcecentre.routledge.com/speechmark

This book is dedicated to Anna Comino-James who asked, "What are you going to do about it?"

CONTENTS

Acknowledgments — *xiv*
Foreword — *xv*

one Introduction — 1
Introduction — *1*
What Is the DME-C Therapy Approach? — *2*
How the DME-C Therapy Approach Came About — *4*
The DME-C Therapy Approach and Its Effectiveness — *6*
Objectives of the Book — *9*
Conclusion — *10*
References — *10*

two High Learning Potential (HLP)/Giftedness — 11
Introduction — *11*
What Are Children with High Learning Potential Like? — *11*
Definition — *11*
Identifying Children with High Learning Potential — *14*
Numbers of Children with High Learning Potential — *15*
Characteristics of Children with High Learning Potential — *15*
Profiles of the Gifted and Talented — *22*
Asynchronous Development — *27*
Dabrowski's Overexcitabilities — *31*
Summary of Needs of Children with High Learning Potential — *35*
Conclusion — *37*
Notes — *37*
References — *37*

three Dual or Multiple Exceptionality (DME)/Twice Exceptionality (2e) — 39
Introduction — *39*
What Is Dual or Multiple Exceptionality (DME) and Twice Exceptionality (2e)? — *39*
How Many Children with DME/2e Are There? — *42*
How to Recognise Children with DME/2e — *42*
Areas of Difficulty in Children with DME/2e — *49*
Barriers that Children with DME/2e Face — *51*
Scenarios of Children with DME/2e — *53*
Support That Children with DME/2e Need — *54*
The Portrayal of DME/2e in the Media — *57*
Well Known People with DME/2e — *58*
Conclusion — *59*
Notes — *59*
References — *60*

Contents

four DME/Twice Exceptionality and Occupational Therapy — 61
- Introduction — 61
- The Non-OT Factors — 63
- A Closer Look at Occupational Therapy for Children in Group 1 – Developmental and Neurological Differences — 67
- Developmental Coordination Disorder (DCD), Including Dyspraxia — 68
- Autism or Autistic Spectrum Disorder (ASD) — 70
- Attention Deficit Hyperactivity Disorder or ADHD — 78
- Conclusion — 83
- Notes — 83
- References — 83

five DME/Twice Exceptionality and Sensory Processing Differences — 86
- Introduction — 86
- Sensory Processing Differences — 86
- Sensory Modulation Disorder — 91
- High Learning Potential and Sensory Processing Differences — 93
- Sensory Based Motor Disorders — 96
- Sensory Discrimination Disorder — 97
- Best Therapy Approach to Help Children with HLP who have Sensory Processing Differences — 97
- Conclusion — 98
- References — 98

six The DME-C Approach's Foundation: The 10 Golden Nuggets — 100
- Introduction — 100
- Questions or Concerns OTs May Have — 100
- The 10 Golden Nuggets — 103
- Conclusion — 127
- Notes — 127
- References — 127

seven The DME-C Approach's Four Walls: The 4 Essential Components — 129
- Introduction — 129
- Essential Component 1: Diarise — 131
- Essential Component 2: Manage transitions — 135
- Essential Component 3: change the Environment and hElp the senses — 139
- Essential Component 4: Communicate — 152
- The 4 Essential Components Working Together — 154
- Conclusion — 154
- Notes — 155
- References — 155

eight Making DME/2e Part of Everyday Occupational Therapy Work — 156
- Introduction — 156
- Evaluation or Assessment — 156
- Report Writing — 157
- Goal Setting — 159
- Re-evaluation — 161
- Further Referral — 162
- Conclusion — 163

nine Case Studies	**164**
Introduction	*164*
Case Study 1: Sally	*167*
Case Study 2: Max	*170*
Case Study 3: Amal	*172*
Case Study 4: Lloyd	*175*
Case Study 5: Imogen	*180*
Case Study 6: Theo	*183*
Case Study 7: Lucas	*186*
Case Study 8: Andy	*189*
Case Study 9: Keli	*192*
Case Study 10: Marco	*195*
Conclusion	*199*
Notes	*199*
References	*199*
ten Resources for Further Help	**200**
Introduction	*200*
UK-based Organisations	*200*
Organisations That Are Accessible from Anywhere	*204*
Organisations in the USA	*206*
Organisations in Australasia	*210*
Glossary	*213*
Index	*220*

ACKNOWLEDGMENTS

Words by Mariza Ferreira:
My heartfelt thanks to my husband Hardus and our two boys Matthew and Josh-Luke for your love, encouragement to follow my passion, and for keeping the cups of coffee coming. To the gifted children with DME/2e and their families who allowed me the privilege of working with them and learning together about what works and what does not. To my colleagues Kirstie, Nikki and Robert who cheered me on over the years. To my fellow paediatric occupational therapists for their enthusiasm and willingness to embark on the journey of helping children with DME/2e with me. To the Royal College of Occupational Therapists Specialist Section Independent Practice, for the Innovation Award to get the book writing process off to the best possible start. To my co-author and friend Rebecca, who thankfully was just as clueless as I was as to what it would take to write this book, or we would have never done it. To my dad Andre who taught me to always give my best and who was so proud of his daughter becoming an author but who passed away before seeing the final product. And lastly to my mum Marie, parents in law Gerhard and Freda and my big sis and lifelong friend Heidi, for all believing in me and carrying me in your prayers.

Words by Rebecca Howell:
It takes such a lot for a book to come to fruition and this one wouldn't have arrived without the help and support of many people. Firstly, thanks to my co-author and friend Mariza, who is fantastic to work with and without whom this book wouldn't be a reality. Thank you to my very good friends Andrea and Pantéa. Andrea for her friendship, discussions and dedication, not only during the writing of the book, but over the past 11 years of sharing family celebrations, holidays, and the highs and lows with one another. Pantéa for her challenging questions, loyal friendship of more years than I care to remember and willingness to pick up where we left off even though years have passed. To Al whom I dance through life with, and who has been there every step of the way. I thank my children, Samuel, Orla and Autumn, whose support and tolerance are wonderful to experience and to witness; these three young people astound me every day. My brother Zack and my sister Adele are, without exception, ready to assist with a listening ear and a helping hand, for which I am truly thankful. To my amazing mum Joyce, who has never put any limit on our abilities and has always encouraged us to reach for our dreams. It doesn't seem right not to mention my late dad Benedict. Although no longer with us, one of his personal philosophies was "If something is worth doing, it is worth getting passionate about". He would be so surprised to see my name on a book. Lastly, the wonderful charity Potential Plus UK that I had personal support from and the privilege to work for, and in particular Julie Taplin whom I enjoyed travelling that journey with and who made many things, including this, possible.

FOREWORD

I have spent my whole working life seeking to maximise the "hidden potential" of children, young people and adults. Nowhere is this more challenging than in helping children and young people (and their parents/carers and the professionals who support them) with DME/2e (or even 3e!). These children are hard to identify; their abilities can disguise their disabilities and the challenges they face (and vice-versa), and they can struggle socially, emotionally and educationally. Moreover, they can often mask either or both their strengths and struggles to attempt to fit in with their peers and to avoid the fates of many who are also neurodivergent, such as becoming victims of bullying or developing mental health issues as a result of misunderstanding, misdiagnosis or lack of appropriate support.

In an inclusive society, both in the classroom and beyond, surely every child and young person has the right to be supported to help maximise their potential and to be recognised and valued for their strengths and abilities, whilst also supported to overcome any challenges they face? Children with DME/2e should not be an exception to this.

Yet we also know that there is a lack of awareness, understanding and approaches to support children and young people who are DME/2e amongst all professionals, including occupational therapists. At best, this presents a risk that traditional interventions will not be effective and at worst the danger of causing harm rather than assistance to those seeking support.

Against this background, every once in a while an approach is developed that can make a significant impact on moving the inclusion debate forward. *Occupational Therapy for Children with DME or Twice Exceptionality* with its DME-C therapy approach does just that for children with DME/2e and who often exist "under the radar" of public and education policy.

We know that many of these children – as well as having amazing abilities and talents – can often be held back by difficulties in areas such as sensory processing, motor coordination, executive functioning and self-regulation. All of these kinds of issues are treated by occupational therapists who, as one parent in the book states, are the "fairy godmothers" (and fathers) of the system, providing the support these children need to unlock their potential.

This is why I believe that *Occupational Therapy for Children with DME or Twice Exceptionality* is a breakthrough book which offers a practical framework and simple steps to both identify dual and multiple exceptionality and supplements current professional OT practice to address appropriately the specific issues these children and young people face.

Both authors have in-depth experience at the "sharp end" of supporting children and young people with DME/2e, and the examples and case studies offered in the book can help occupational therapists adapt and extend their work to support DME/2e. Not only that, but I believe that every professional across the practice spectrum, parent/carer and teacher should be aware of the approach outlined in this book. Used in the right way, it could have a major impact on issues ranging from school phobia to behavioural issues at home or in the classroom; mental health challenges to issues related to underachievement and beyond.

We do not know how many children with DME there are in the UK; 80,000 is a conservative estimate and there could be many more. Imagine the impact on the wellbeing of our children if even half of these could engage in and benefit from the approach outlined in this book?

Denise Yates MBE, author of *Parenting Dual Exceptional Children* and co-author of *The School Handbook for Dual and Multiple Exceptionality*

Chapter one

Introduction

Introduction

It is estimated that there are about 60,000 to 80,000 children in England and Wales alone who have dual or multiple exceptionality (DME)[1,2] or twice exceptionality (2e). The former term is the one currently in use in the UK and was first introduced in a series of government documents on gifted and talented education in 2008.[3] The latter term is the one used across most of the world, including the USA and Australia. One of the most widely accepted definitions for dual or multiple exceptionality in the UK is:

> In the gifted education field, 2e and DME are terms to describe those who are intellectually very able (gifted) or who have a talent (a special gift in a performance or skill area) and in addition to this have a special educational need
>
> *(Montgomery 2015).*

According to this definition, a child who is considered to be intellectually gifted can have exceptional potential and/or ability with regards to academic subjects, and/or a child can be exceptionally talented in other areas such as sports or the arts, e.g. acting or playing a musical instrument. The bottom line is that their ability in that particular area is much more advanced compared to their peers.

Sometimes children who are intellectually able or talented also have a special educational need, learning difference or disability that makes it difficult for them to reach their full potential. The term "special educational need" or SEND ("special educational need and disability"), as it is more commonly known in the UK, includes a whole range of needs or challenges such as dyslexia, autism, sensory processing differences, developmental coordination disorder (DCD) including dyspraxia and attention deficit hyperactivity disorder or ADHD, although there are many more. Lots of children have more than one diagnosis. For example, a child may have high cognitive ability but also handwriting difficulties as part of developmental coordination disorder, making it difficult to evidence their knowledge and learning through writing. It is therefore possible that an intellectually gifted child could have a SEND that severely impacts their ability to achieve at the level they would otherwise be capable of and could achieve with the right support. Or, a child may be an exceptional tennis player and autistic, meaning that they have difficulties interacting with other players on the court, impacting their ability to practise their hitting skills with others. In each case where a child has a gift or talent as well as a special educational need and/or disability, they would be viewed as having the profile of dual or multiple exceptionality (DME) or twice exceptionality (2e).

DOI: 10.4324/9781003334033-1

2 Introduction

Paediatric occupational therapists are some of the best-suited professionals to help children with DME/2e, particularly gifted (or high learning potential/HLP) children who have sensory processing differences, motor coordination difficulties, and concentration difficulties as well as executive functioning (and self-regulation) difficulties impacting their activity participation. This is because of the unique training occupational therapists undergo, which has a holistic focus on approaching a child's difficulties to engage in relevant tasks. Occupational therapists consider a child's physical, mental, social, emotional and environmental barriers and use various therapy approaches and techniques to address these. However, where children with DME/2e are concerned, it is essential to understand the strengths and weaknesses of their individual profiles as well as use techniques that deviate from the traditional way of providing occupational therapy to be effective and achieve favourable outcomes. This is confirmed by various international articles[4,5,6,7] that promote occupational therapy as being generally beneficial for HLP/gifted/DME/2e children and acknowledge that it needs to be adapted for them. However, very little guidance has been given on how to go about providing a suitably adapted approach. Hence the creation of the DME-C therapy approach.

What Is the DME-C Therapy Approach?

The therapy approach for helping dual or multiple exceptional children, or the DME-C therapy approach, is a practical guide to support paediatric occupational therapists in their one-to-one work with children with DME/2e who have challenges specifically relating to sensory processing, unhelpful thought patterns and self-regulation. Furthermore, it also contains guidance on how therapists can approach therapy (the method) when addressing other challenges that children with DME/2e may face which impact their occupational performance and are not necessarily rooted in sensory processing differences. The approach caters to the needs of children with DME/2e in a way that traditional approaches do not, as it actively considers HLP and DME/2e as part of a child's presentation to inform therapy.

The DME-C therapy approach is not intended for implementation in a group setting. While many occupational therapy approaches are very effective, and in fact often rely on being provided in group format, it is not the case with the DME-C therapy approach. This is because, in our experience of working with children with HLP or giftedness and DME/2e, the treating therapist needs to maintain a high level of observation and awareness of the child during sessions in order to guide sessions appropriately; something that is difficult to achieve otherwise. However, there are some isolated cases where therapy can be provided for two children at the same time, but this is under very specific circumstances and only if the therapist has given the option careful consideration. For example, we have successfully treated siblings who were close in age, generally got along well, exhibited the same type of challenges and were able to learn from and support each other during therapy.

The DME-C therapy approach can roughly be compared to a basic house, which has a foundation and four walls. For a building to be strong, safe and ultimately habitable, the foundation and walls have to comply with strict building regulations (yes, we know there is a lot

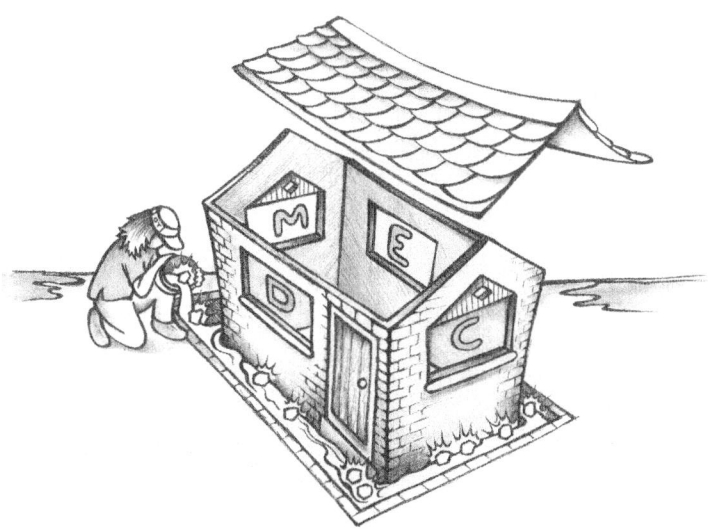

more to it). However, how the builders or interior decorators decide to furnish the house internally, is up to them. Similarly, the DME-C therapy approach relies heavily on having a strong foundation (the 10 Golden Nuggets) and walls (the 4 Essential Components) which comply with specific guidance, but how occupational therapists decide to furnish it inside (deciding which activities to use), is up to them. Lastly, we view the authenticity that the therapist brings to the therapy process as the "roof" that covers the house or compliments the whole therapy process.

The DME-C therapy approach's foundation and four walls are equally important. The raw materials that make up its **foundation**, the 10 Golden Nuggets, are the **ten key factors** an occupational therapist working with children with DME/2e should build into their **method of providing therapy**, discussed in Chapter 6. It relates to the non-OT factors (see Chapter 4), and we are convinced that it has a significant impact on successful therapy outcomes, not just for children with DME/2e who have sensory processing differences, unhelpful thought patterns and self-regulation challenges, but also those who have other SENDs which we discuss in Chapter 4 as well as other occupational performance challenges that may not fit into any of these mentioned categories.

The **four walls** of the approach are the 4 Essential Components that should be addressed in the therapy provision for a child with DME/2e and sensory processing differences, unhelpful thought patterns and self-regulation challenges. Each component is represented by a different letter as below:

- D for Diarise
- M for Manage transitions

- E for change the Environment and hElp the senses
- C for Communicate

Why 10 Golden Nuggets and 4 Essential components? Well, when gold miners dig for gold they have to unearth large amounts of soil and sift through it using various methods, from gold pans to large wash plant machines, in order to get to the gold. Finding "what works best" with children with DME/2e was a little like this and it took a lot of moving ground to find the golden nuggets – the methods of providing or presenting therapy that transformed our work with children with DME/2e. Similarly, the four walls are the essential components we found that needed to be included in therapy for the best possible chance of success. Although we have used the letters D, M, E and C for their similarity to **D**ual or **M**ultiple **E**xceptional **C**hildren to represent the 4 Essential Components, these four components **have to** be combined with the 10 Golden Nuggets to make up the full DME-C therapy approach.

We want to be clear that the DME-C therapy approach is **not** a therapy program with set activities to be followed from first to last session in a rigid way, and that any examples of activities we give throughout this book are by way of explanation only to achieve the 4 Essential Components of Diarise, Manage transitions, change the Environment and hElp the senses, and Communicate. We believe that, just like the children we treat are unique, each occupational therapist is unique in their skills set and what they have to offer children with DME/2e. Occupational therapists can therefore draw on their own knowledge and experience of activities and through the process of activity analysis, determine if the activities are in line with the guidance of the approach and/or whether they need some adjusting. This is the "internal furnishing of the house" we referred to earlier.

How the DME-C Therapy Approach Came About

Words by Rebecca, former director of the DME Trust and senior education consultant at Potential Plus UK:

While working at the charity Potential Plus UK, in conjunction with my colleague Radhika Rajbans, I set up the charity's assessment service in 2013. We soon found that lots of children who were coming to us had some challenges alongside their advanced abilities. These challenges were impacting their lives, stopping them participating in activities and preventing them from realising their potential. Our research, understanding and experience led us to include a questionnaire about sensory processing early in the service's development, and we were surprised to find that over 50% of the children we assessed had some sensory processing problems. Once we had identified these, however, we wanted to be able to signpost the children and their families to further support this.

I first met Mariza through a mutual friend and, knowing she was a well-respected paediatric occupational therapist, we agreed to meet to discuss the matter. Mariza was approachable, engaging and open-minded. I knew at once that I could work with her! Initially, we shared notes. I told Mariza about the children with high learning potential and DME/2e who we worked with. Mariza shared with me and my team how occupational therapy could support such children and gave pointers for how parents could best support children with sensory processing problems. As our collaboration grew, Mariza ran several sessions for parents and our assessors who referred families to her. Mariza developed her expertise in working with children with DME/2e over several years of our collaboration.

As Mariza's experience of working with children with high learning potential and DME/2e grew, so did her involvement in networks in the field. She took part in several conferences funded by The Potential Trust and in 2017 we went together to a round-table meeting in Oslo, Norway to talk about how occupational therapists could help these children. She also talked about the topic in occupational therapy networks and conferences.

Not only did the demand for Mariza's services outstrip her capacity, many families were in different geographical areas and so could not access her therapy. In addition, we realised that the more occupational therapists who knew about children with high learning potential and DME/2e, the more children could be supported to thrive where they were currently struggling. We were on a mission to spread the word and so, with the support of Anna Comino-James, a trustee of The Potential Trust, we started to plan our first professional development opportunity for occupational therapists.

Words by Mariza, occupational therapist:

It was never the intention to create a new therapy approach when I started to work with children with high learning potential or giftedness, who were struggling with activity participation due to "sensory issues" and "difficulties controlling their emotions", which were the most common reasons they sought therapy. Rather, it was the product of a therapist desperate to help a group of children for whom the traditional way of providing and delivering therapy did not seem to work as well as it did for children with the same issues, but who were not considered to have DME/2e. This was a group of children who, despite their abundant potential, were not reaching it academically and/or socially because of barriers which seemed to extend beyond those mentioned above.

Going back to the drawing board, I made a conscious effort to learn more about the profiles and needs of children with high learning potential and DME/2e. I wanted to be clear in my own mind which areas of difficulty I was able to address, which ones I could not and how I could more effectively address the issues that fell within my remit or scope as an occupational therapist. I gave things a go, communicating to the children with DME/2e and their families that I was trialling different ways of working, and that we needed to work together to achieve our therapy goals. I started noticing some recurring themes that needed to be addressed in therapy, which ultimately led to the creation of the DME-C approach.

Colleagues thought me "brave", which in the UK actually means crazy, to even attempt a new way of working. But I had an intense desire to help the highly gifted children and their families who came my way. I was also self-employed, so my income was dependent on successful therapy outcomes as without them I would not get further referrals.

I have been in the fortunate position to have co-trained over 30 UK based therapists in the DME-C therapy approach between 2019 and 2021 with Rebecca Howell, who at the time was the senior educational consultant at Potential Plus UK, a national charity that supports children with high learning potential and DME/2e, and director of The DME Trust. We called the course, "Occupational Therapy for Children with HLP and DME/2e" or OT4DME in short. It was, in fact, understanding the needs of occupational therapists working with children with DME/2e through running these courses that inspired us to write this book so that we can reach even more professionals and therefore more children, as our goal has and always will be to support children with DME/2e the best we can.

I am passionate about improving the lives of children with high learning potential and DME/2e, and have no doubt that occupational therapy is the vital link for helping them reach their potential. I believe that through my work I can change the world one child at a time. And I am taking as many occupational therapists, other child professionals and parents as possible on this journey with me.

The DME-C Therapy Approach and Its Effectiveness

We know that the DME-C therapy approach works because of the quantitative and qualitative evidence collected over the years. This came through formal feedback forms completed by the parents and carers of children with DME/2e who were treated using the DME-C therapy approach (and sometimes the children themselves) and occupational therapists who attended our OT4DME courses and use the principles of the DME-C therapy approach in their work with children with DME/2e. Additional evidence is regularly gathered informally as parents and therapists contact us to report on the positive effect of the DME-C therapy approach.

Parents consistently rate the DME-C therapy approach as highly effective for their children (nine or ten on a scale of one to ten). All the therapists (100%) who attended the OT4DME courses, rated it as "excellent" and stated that they moved from knowing nothing about DME/2e (one on a scale of one to five) to knowing a lot about DME/2e (four or five on a scale of one to five). Furthermore, 97% of therapists stated they strongly agreed that they would use a combination of the 10 Golden Nuggets and 4 Essential Components in their future work with children with DME/2e. Also, in a follow up survey, 83% of therapists who responded strongly agreed that the DME-C therapy approach made them better at their jobs (four or five on a scale of one to five)

Below we have listed a selection of parent/carer and child feedback, followed by some comments made by occupational therapists. Please note that further parent/carer and child feedback is listed throughout this book and especially in Chapter 9 where we discuss ten case studies to illustrate how the DME-C therapy approach was used in treatment.

Parent/carer and child feedback

Here are some of the amazing comments we have had from parents, carers and children:

> "The therapy sessions were literally life-saving for my child. It was not a 'one size fits all' approach, which is the same for all children. I felt that the therapy was specific to my child's needs and she felt that too".
>
> (Parent)

> "It was such a relief to find a professional that understood and valued my child's sensitivity and learning style. This meant that the sessions were an enjoyable experience (I think I learnt as much as my child!). There was a really comprehensive approach to ways of dealing with the sensitive hearing issue – both sensory and thought processes. I loved the way the therapist adapted sessions according to my child's reactions. He is now much more confident about coping with his sensitive hearing, and also has learnt to be better at making his voice heard if things are not okay. The sessions have confirmed my suspicions that occupational therapists are actually the fairy godmothers of this world, and everyone should be assigned one at birth".
>
> (Parent)

> "Assemblies and lessons go so much quicker now. Whereas before I would have been fidgeting and restless, now I feel like I'm much more settled. I looked at my watch in maths and thought I had been there about ten minutes but actually we were forty minutes in. At the beginning of term, mega assembly, which goes on for an hour and usually feels like five hours, this time felt like ten minutes. I think this is because of the sensory obstacle courses I now do in the morning before school that I learnt about in occupational therapy".
>
> (Child with DME/2e)

> "Therapy sessions were very practical and helped my child to help herself. Signposting to autism was also very useful, and she has since been diagnosed as autistic. The therapist's understanding of DME/2e was extremely helpful as my child is exceptionally good at masking, but the therapist treated her exactly right for an autistic child with extremely high intelligence".
>
> (Parent)

> "We feel so lucky that, between the school SENDCO, form teachers, Potential Plus UK and the occupational therapist, our daughter (KF) has received wonderful support and understanding along the way. Together we have been able to piece together so many parts of the 'KF puzzle' and get her to what I think will be a good place to start secondary school".
>
> (Parent)

Occupational therapists' feedback

Here are some of the overwhelmingly positive comments we have had from occupational therapists:

"The OT4DME training was informative and inspirational. It opened up my view of DME/2e and the role of the OT".

"The DME-C approach has been put together in a simple yet creative way. It allows the child with DME/2e to differentiate themselves in a practical way and learn to work **with** their differences instead of being taken over or ruled by it".

"I will be able to immediately implement the ideas presented in my practice to help support and unblock some of my clients in their therapeutic journeys".

"I am feeling really inspired and cannot wait to embed some of the ideas from the DME-C approach in my practice to be able to help local families get the support they need".

"I am now thinking of my caseload kids in a different light and will be reflecting on what I will be doing differently with potential DME kids".

"While attending the training I had an 'aha' moment – identifying certain clients that I have not been able to understand and who responded well to sensory integration therapy but who struggled with emotional regulation. I knew that something was going on, just not what!".

"I loved the practical examples of how to work differently with children with DME/2e, it was an eye opener".

"The examples of activities are very useful to build on".

"I particularly enjoyed discussing how to help this special group of children for whom there is so little understanding and provision".

"I feel like I am leaving the training with so much practical advice that is both motivating and enabling".

"I came away feeling totally inspired and excited about occupational therapy again".

"I left the OT4DME course so motivated that I contacted a past client's mum to encourage her to look into DME/2e as I suspected her son fits into this category".

"The OT4DME course and the knowledge I gained, enabled me to support a child for further referral (to assess their cognitive ability) and subsequent correct identification of having the profile of DME/2e. The parents provided positive feedback about the process and the focussed support their child received in school as a result. Their lives have improved significantly".

"Since learning more about DME/2e, I assessed a child who I suspected had DME/2e. I adapted my assessment and printed off advanced science and maths worksheets, which were his interests, and used these to assess his writing, visual motor integration, etc".

"The knowledge of DME/2e has helped me to identify children with DME/2e during the assessment process which has been crucial. When I now meet these children, I know how important it is that they are understood. My recommendations in their reports have strongly encouraged a strength-based approach amongst many other bits of information that signposts them and their family to resources that are available. While I have used some of the Golden Nuggets in therapy, such as designing unexpected or delayed outcomes, it has been part of my Sensory Integration Therapy approach, using Ayres Sensory Integration. One kid had the answers, but needed help with using strategies when anxiety got in his way just before transitions. He developed his own sensory ladder to use at home and at school with an adult to help him. Throughout sessions, he was able to identify that he gave up very easily when something did not 'go his way', and this was something that he was able to work on and develop. This child was also doing incredible extra-curricular activities, such as Mandarin, and it was important to signpost him to groups that were available to support equally gifted children of his age so that there was a sense of social participation, and also an essence of fun. The continuing problem would remain that he was brighter than his teachers which he was fully aware of, and this would mean monitoring and education of teaching staff about DME/2e – something I had to make the school SENCO aware of".

(Feedback summarised)

Objectives of the Book

The main objectives of this book are for paediatric occupational therapists to:

1. Learn what it means when children are referred to as having the profile of DME/2e, and how to recognise when children have DME/2e
2. Understand the issues children with DME/2e have which do not directly relate to the remit or scope of occupational therapy but which are essential to consider in therapy (the non-OT factors)
3. Understand the main SEND (special educational need or disabilities) or learning differences that children with DME/2e have
4. Understand the foundation (the 10 Golden Nuggets) and four walls (the 4 Essential Components) of the DME-C therapy approach to guide their work with children with DME/2e who have sensory processing differences, unhelpful thought patterns and who struggle with some aspects of executive functioning (emotional self-regulation), to ensure effective therapy outcomes
5. Be presented with example activities to use in therapy to achieve the principles of the DME-C therapy approach with children with DME/2e and their families, and also a suggested therapy progression plan
6. Read case studies to learn how to apply their understanding
7. Understand how to implement the DME-C foundation or 10 Golden Nuggets in their approach to therapy with children with DME/2e regardless of their SEND or learning difference

8. Know where to access more information and support in their work with children with DME/2e
9. Know where to signpost children with DME/2e and their families with regards to needs which fall outside of the occupational therapy remit or scope

Conclusion

Many paediatric occupational therapists that we have worked with tell us they have encountered children that fit the profile of DME/2e in the course of their work but without knowing it at the time. On reflection, they confirmed that traditional therapy approaches, while not entirely unsuccessful, did not have the same effects as with other children, which mirrors our own initial experiences of working with and observing children with DME/2e, until we developed the effective approach that we offer in this book.

We also come across many paediatric occupational therapists who report they had no idea that children with DME/2e existed or how to help them. In view of the large number of children across the world who have a DME/2e profile, we are on a mission to empower occupational therapists to be aware of how to support this group of children. Writing this book is one of the ways we are doing that.

References

1 Potential Plus UK (2019) *F01 Dual or Multiple Exceptionality* [Fact Sheet].
2 Ryan, A. & Waterman, C. (2018) *Dual and Multiple Exceptionality: The Current State of Play*. nasen.
3 Department for Children, Schools and Families. 2008: *Gifted and Talented Education, helping to find and support children with dual or multiple exceptionalities*. Nottingham: DCSF Publications.
4 Gere, D., Capps, S.,Mitchell, D., & Grubbs, E. (2009). Sensory sensitivities of gifted children. *The American Journal of Occupational Therapy*, 63(3), 288-295.
5 Jarrard, P. (2008) *Sensory Issues in Gifted Children: Synthesis of the Literature*, retrieved from: https://sensoryhealth.org/sites/default/files/publications/SensoryissuesinGiftedChildren.pdf.
6 Johnson, D. (2012) *Occupational Therapy and Twice-Exceptional Students*, article in 2e Newsletter Sept/Oct 2012, retrieved from http://www.2enewsletter.com/subscribers_only/arch_2012_09_johnson.html.
7 Ochsenbein, M. (2019) *Working with Twice Exceptional Clients*, article in May 2019 Education Newsletter on STAR Institute website, retrieved from https://sensoryhealth.org/basic/may-2019-education-newsletter.

Chapter two
High Learning Potential (HLP)/Giftedness

Introduction

This chapter is an introduction to what high learning potential, or giftedness, is and how occupational therapists can start to recognise children with this trait. It discusses the definitions of children with high learning potential, the characteristics of these children and their common profiles. The chapter introduces the concepts of asynchronous development and overexcitabilities as foundations for discussions on DME/2e, sensory processing differences and self-regulation difficulties in the rest of the book.

What Are Children with High Learning Potential Like?

Have you come across a child whose advanced vocabulary surprises you? Is there a child who has brought a thick chapter book with a complex plot to a therapy session? Have you met a child who seemingly knows all there is to know about stars and planets? What about one who could talk about the science of rainbows? Maybe you have come across a child who wanted to know a lot about the fixtures and fittings in your therapy room. Was there a time when a child seemed to pick up everything you were teaching very quickly and wanted to move on before even you were ready? Have you come across a child who had a very advanced ability with numbers and was able to add up or multiply large numbers in their head? Have you been astounded by a child's amazing artistic ability? Have you met a child who has an intense interest and ability in playing the violin? It is possible that these children were gifted, or had high learning potential (HLP). Usually, when children demonstrate some advanced abilities for their age, as in the snapshots above, it is a sign that they have high cognitive ability that not only can be applied to areas of learning but pervades all their life experiences. It is important that therapists recognise this is part of a child's profile so they can adjust their practice and accommodate all their differences. Not all children who have high learning potential will show it in such obvious ways as outlined above. With some, it will take time and the development of a rapport with the therapist before these children will be comfortable enough to demonstrate their abilities.

Definition

High learning potential, or giftedness, in children generally means that the child has some cognitive abilities that are significantly advanced for their age. These cognitive abilities may be generalised, such as having a high IQ, or specific, such as visuospatial skills. Giftedness is a form of neurodivergence, meaning that people who have high learning potential tend

DOI: 10.4324/9781003334033-2

to have a set of characteristics different to neurotypical people. It also means that people with high learning potential tend to experience the world differently to neurotypical people.

The term high learning potential, as opposed to giftedness, first started to be used in the UK in the mid-2010s when the national charity Potential Plus UK adopted it as their preferred term to describe children who were traditionally referred to as gifted. This came after much debate and years of misunderstanding about the term gifted, which tends to give a false impression that those with abilities significantly beyond the expected for their age have a gift that they can use without experiencing difficulties or challenges. The newer term acknowledges that, in children particularly, giftedness is about the potential for achievements. It also acknowledges that not everyone has the optimum conditions or support to utilise their innate abilities, although society often still looks to performance or achievements for evidence of high ability, such as in a school context. The term high learning potential can be, and is, used interchangeably for the term gifted. We use both terms throughout this book.

Whilst there is no universal definition of what it means to be gifted or have high learning potential,[1] some of the most common definitions state that gifted individuals have cognitive abilities within the top 2% of the population and others put this figure within the top 5%. Experts and practitioners dealing with children who have advanced abilities do need vocabulary to talk about what the right support and accommodations are for them, and it is generally recognised that what this group of children need in terms of handling, provision and accommodations may be very different to what is currently the standard offer for all children.

It is important to bear in mind there is no particular cut-off point that makes a person gifted or not since it depends very much on their profile, background and opportunities. One example of this is that a child may have certain challenges which get in the way of them being able to perform in a test, and so they may score lower than expected given their character traits. Another example is that a child may come from a family who ridicules the demonstration of their abilities, and so they have learned not to show them. This means that a child scoring below the 5% range mentioned above in a test of cognitive abilities is not necessarily not gifted; a professional would look at the child's profile, background and other evidence to add into the mix. In particular, it is well-documented that autistic children underperform on traditional IQ tests due to the reliance on language skills, ability to interact with others, motor planning and execution (part of dyspraxia), as some tests require recreating shapes with manipulatives and behavioural regulation (specifically the ability to sit still and focus for the required amount of time to complete the tests).[2]

For the purposes of this book and in line with Potential Plus UK's guidance, we present and subscribe to Prof. Steven Pfeiffer's Tripartite Model of Giftedness[3] to underpin our work. We feel this is a fairer way to view the subject and prevent unnecessary and harmful barriers being put in the way of those needing support due to their high learning potential/giftedness. The Tripartite Model of Giftedness conceptualises high learning potential/giftedness in an inclusive way, offering multiple ways of perceiving those who have significantly advanced abilities.

High Learning Potential (HLP)/Giftedness 13

The three perspectives within the Tripartite Model of Giftedness are giftedness viewed through a lens of high intelligence, giftedness viewed through a lens of outstanding accomplishments and giftedness viewed through a lens of potential to excel. An individual need not fit into each of these three categories, nor are they mutually exclusive.

High intelligence

In the first of these three perspectives – giftedness viewed through a lens of high intelligence – high learning potential is usually identified through some sort of cognitive ability test. These may be administered through a school, such as CAT tests or non-verbal reasoning tests, or during an individual assessment that may have been sought out privately to discover more about a child's learning profile, such as those carried out by Potential Plus UK, an educational psychologist or part of a diagnosis pathway. Scores within the top of the above average range and above, i.e. the top 5%, usually indicate that a child should be viewed as gifted/high learning potential through this lens.

Outstanding accomplishments

In the second of the three perspectives – giftedness through a lens of outstanding accomplishments – the model considers the achievements of the individual as compared to other children their age. This is usually through academics in a school context, and academic excellence is the defining characteristic here, where high learning potential/giftedness can

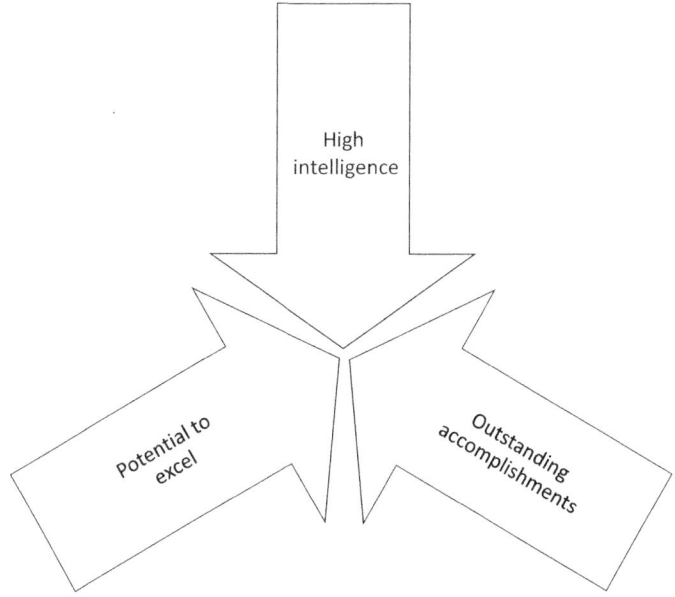

Figure 2.1 The Tripartite Model of Giftedness, Prof. Steven Pfeiffer.

be identified through the tracking of the child's academic performance and the results of tests. However, this is not necessarily across the board as creativity, motivation, persistence and academic passion are also important characteristics, since they play a large role in success, and can be discussed and identified.

Potential to excel

The final perspective is giftedness through a lens of potential to excel. This last category exists because some young people do not have sufficient opportunity to develop latent talents or demonstrate what they are capable of. Not all young people start out on an equal footing and it takes access to resources, time and encouragement to develop abilities even in the most talented of individuals. It also exists because there are some groups who are unable to be tested, such as those with a visual or auditory sensory impairment, and some who regularly underachieve, such as those who are disadvantaged, those who are young and bilingual, those with cultural differences and those who are neurodivergent. This group is the most difficult to identify, but it is essential that therapists and other professionals are on the lookout for those who fit into this category so they can be provided with the opportunities and accommodations they need to realise their potential. Children who fall into this category are often recognised by parents, teachers and other professionals as quick learners, highly curious and as understanding complex concepts despite the socio-economic, language, cultural or disability-related challenges they have. In these cases, determining whether they have high learning potential needs to be looked at holistically and by taking into account background information, characteristics of the child, their cognitive, physical and social development, etc.

Identifying Children with High Learning Potential

The children who are definitely within the gifted bracket are those who have had tests and scored in one or more areas of cognitive ability (IQ) or achievement (usually maths, reading, spelling, writing) in the top 5%, on or above 95th percentile, for their age. Whether or not this means they need something different in terms of education and provision depends on the individual child and their profile, but they usually need some adjustment (since the regular curriculum is unlikely to meet their educational needs) where the scores are in the top 2%, or on or above the 98th percentile. However, scores that are within the top 2% are difficult to be accurate about, and the higher the scores the more this is true. This is because when tests are being designed, usually around 150 individuals are tested in each age band (more than this only improves accuracy slightly over the whole range), so only two to three children tested will have scored within the top 2% of each age band. This is why some tests have "extended norms", meaning they have been tested on more individuals at the top end, so that they can be more accurate at the higher extreme.

Another strong sign that a child has high learning potential is when they have demonstrated that they are capable of working consistently more than one year ahead of their peers in at least one area of academic performance. A child who is reading and understanding books that are well beyond the expectation for their age would be an example of this. Another would be a child who is excelling in maths (in the understanding of concepts as well as being able to calculate ahead of their age) in school. Additionally, when a child shows signs that they might have high learning potential, such as those mentioned in the first section of this chapter or some of the characteristics discussed later, professionals should look at the child's full profile to consider whether giftedness might be part of their profile. Identifying children who have both high learning potential and a special educational need or disability, called dual or multiple exceptional (DME)/twice exceptional (2e), can be trickier and will be discussed more fully in Chapters 3 and 4.

Numbers of Children with High Learning Potential

There are more than 1.5 million children with high learning potential in the UK, which is 10% of the population from 0 to 19 years of age.[4] This figure is based on including children from the three groups of the Tripartite Model and is in line with the definition of "high attainers" by the Sutton Trust[5] and England's former Department of Children Schools and Families guidance for identifying gifted and talented learners.[6] Of these, approximately 313,000 children will have exceptionally high cognitive abilities and be in the top 2% of the population. Furthermore, 70,600 children with high learning potential are born each year in the UK, which is 10% of the total new births. Whilst they are in a minority, these are quite large figures that demonstrate there is certainly demand for bespoke services to support children with high learning potential.

Across all schools in the UK, approximately one million children have high learning potential, representing 10% of the school population in children of compulsory school age (5 to 16 years old) and including young people from the three groups of the Tripartite Model.

Characteristics of Children with High Learning Potential

Although children with high learning potential are a diverse group, there are some characteristics that are common amongst them. First and foremost, and by definition, the most common characteristic that almost all high learning potential children share is that they learn quickly. This does not necessarily mean they will learn everything quickly; everyone is motivated by different things, and some have barriers to learning in certain areas, particularly where there is a special educational need or learning difference involved. Often, this ability to absorb information is accompanied by being able to understand complex concepts and retain information, i.e. a good long-term memory.

Linda Silverman's Characteristics of Giftedness Scale[7] identifies 25 characteristics that are commonly reported by parents of children with IQ scores over 120. Indeed, "learns rapidly" and "excellent memory" are two of the characteristics mentioned there. The checklist also refers to gifted children having an extensive vocabulary, reasoning well, having strong curiosity, having a mature sense of humour and keen observation. Other characteristics mentioned are a compassion for others, perfectionism, a vivid imagination, a long attention span (for their age), ability with numbers, concern with justice and fairness, sensitivity and a wide range of interests. How these characteristics commonly present in our experience is explained in more detail below with everyday examples and pseudonyms used to aid understanding. Work has been done on how signs of giftedness present in different cultures and the 15 characteristics (a subset of the Characteristics of Giftedness Scale) below are identified across the world.[8]

Learns rapidly

The defining characteristic, rapid assimilation of information in at least one area, is something that all children with HLP have in common. This does not necessarily mean they will learn rapidly in all areas, but they are very likely to in areas of interest and the things they pay attention to. Some may have relative difficulties learning in some areas (such as a dyslexic learner in spelling).

> **Example:**
>
> Preschool keyworker Adele Huntley is astounded by a child in her group, Maia, who is three years old. Maia comes to nursery every week having progressed significantly with not just reading and maths knowledge, but knowledge and understanding of the world. In just a few weeks she has gone from starting to sound out words to reading sentences in starter books fluently and with expression. In the same timeframe, she has progressed from recognising the numbers one to ten to now being able to name numbers up to 100. Each time a new topic is introduced, Maia already has some knowledge of it and comes to nursery the next time with even more facts or understanding she has learned in the interim.

Excellent long-term memory

Many children with HLP are able to remember information easily. There seems to be a well-trodden path to their long-term memories, meaning that what they pay attention to (and sometimes information they get in passing) is remembered and built upon later (sometimes much later).

> **Example:**
>
> Teacher Phil Harwood had a seven-year-old child with HLP, Juniper, in his Year 3 class. He observed that Juniper would often already know what was being taught, for example in topic work like "the Romans". When he quizzed her on how she knew things, she would answer that she had read a book on the topic some years previously or she had

visited a museum and read about it there. He found he had to adapt the learning opportunities for Juniper so she could extend her knowledge and understanding.

Extensive vocabulary

This ability to learn quickly and remember information means that many children with HLP pick up vocabulary, easily resulting in an extensive vocabulary. There are exceptions to this such as in young bilingual children or in neurodivergent populations.

Example:

In occupational therapist Jodie Knowles' practice, one of the children she was treating was six-year-old Henry. Jodie was blown away by the vocabulary Henry knew and used in a casual manner. He would regularly use phrases such as "insatiable thirst", "fortunate timing" and "of my own volition".

Reasons well

Another contributing factor for why children with HLP learn so rapidly is that they are able to draw inferences or conclusions from the facts they know.[9] This kind of reasoning is applied to fill gaps in knowledge or come up with surprising solutions. It also means they can often put forward well-reasoned arguments in a discussion. As Kanevsky puts it, reasoning well in gifted children is an "outstanding ability to think things through and consider implications or alternatives; rich, flexible, highly conscious, logical thought".[10]

Example:

Two-year-old Magali's mother is often in awe at her daughter's ability to reason. Magali easily recalls things that happened the previous day, week and month and can understand where they fit in a timeline. She uses this recall to solve problems that come up, such as her mother wondering where to post a letter when out one day. Magali remembered that they had posted a letter in a letterbox just around the corner a couple of months beforehand and suggested it to her mother.

Strong curiosity

Because of their clarity of understanding of the world, many children with HLP want to further that understanding and find out more.[11] If they are confident and are in a situation to be able to ask, this is likely to be demonstrated through asking questions about the things they are interested in. Others may gain new understanding through books, documentaries and the like, amazing adults around them with their quest for knowledge.

> **Example:**
>
> Six-year-old Sam is fascinated by anything to do with computers. He has exhausted his parents' understanding about the topic and watches endless YouTube videos about it. He has taught himself to do basic coding and talks about quantum computing to anyone who will listen.

Mature sense of humour

Children with HLP often have a sense of humour[12] that is advanced for their age. In fact, some say that this is often the first or tell-tale sign of a child being gifted. The reason for this ability is that children with high learning potential are able to understand ambiguity, hidden meanings and idioms; parts of speech that are often used in humour.

> **Example:**
>
> Two-year-old Precious astounds her father with her ability to play on words at such a young age. One day she asked her father if he wanted a bear hug. When her father said yes, she ran to get her comically oversized teddy bear and gave it to him to hug. Her father hugged the bear and said thank you. Precious replied, "you're bear-y welcome"!

Keen observation

The natural curiosity and ability to reason well in children with HLP means they are often keen observers of the world. They want to know more and observe so they can notice patterns and categorise things in a way that makes sense to them.

> **Example:**
>
> Gabby is ten years old and has a passion for the natural world. She keeps notebooks in which she records her studies of bugs and other wildlife in the garden. She recognises different species of beetle through her observations and cross-referencing to books her parents have bought her. Gabby would like to be an entomologist when she grows up.

Compassion for others

Many children with HLP have an emotional sensitivity that leads them to have a compassion for others, manifesting in getting upset when hearing about bad things happening locally and around the world or watching films/TV programmes that have a human story in them.

Example:

Daniele is eleven years old and often gets scared or upset by things he watches on TV. His friends all enjoy watching Dr Who but Daniele really struggles with the disasters that befall people in the programme. He thinks everyone should have a secure home and is passionate about fundraising for homelessness and water-aid causes. He spends some weekends baking cakes to sell to raise money for these charities at events.

Perfectionism

Children with HLP tend to experience perfectionism, becoming upset or anxious when their efforts are not up to their self-imposed standards. When children with HLP are young, they tend to experience success at learning many things easily. This, combined with an acute understanding of what adult-level achievement looks like in many domains, leads to the feelings of frustration they have when they are unable to meet this benchmark, even though they would not be expected to achieve at this level due to their age and development.

Example:

Nine-year-old Jamie is a very keen artist and produces very technical drawings that show an ability well beyond his age level. However, in his mind's eye, Jamie knows what he wants his drawing to come out like and gets frustrated when he cannot produce what he can imagine. He has been known to tear up almost-finished drawings, swipe his drawing equipment off the table, storm out of the room, cry loudly in anger and frustration and shout at his family at these times.

Vivid imagination

Many children with HLP have very vivid imaginations that show through role play and giving personalities to toys when they are little. This can also be the source of some anxiety for them since they can imagine the outcomes of situations and may lack the life experience to understand how likely perceived negative outcomes are.

Example:

Fran is eight years old and plays many role play games in which she makes up characters and scenarios. When she was younger, she had a pretend friend called Coco who

> still makes an "appearance" occasionally. Her current passion is making up plays and musicals for her puppet theatre and acting them out to her family.

Long attention span

Especially when they are young, many children with HLP demonstrate a very long attention span compared to their peers. They may show remarkable persistence in the areas they are interested in, and this contributes to how quickly they learn.

> **Example:**
>
> Jacques is two years old. His nursery keyworker is amazed by how long he stays at tasks like colouring, artwork and "experiments" in the sand pit and water tray. Even if he is interrupted for a mealtime he goes straight back to what he was doing before until he has completed his task.

Ability with numbers

Many children with HLP have an early fondness for numbers and enjoy the logical way they work. They are often able to perform calculations well beyond the expectation for their age and understand advanced mathematical concepts. Some gifted children have an extremely advanced facility with numbers. Some also extend their fondness for numbers into other areas of their lives, like enjoying reading anything to do with numbers such as the *Murderous Maths* books and involving numbers in role play scenarios.

> **Example:**
>
> Amna is four years old and has just started school. Her teacher is blown away by her ability with numbers. She can count into the thousands, add together double-digit numbers and multiple single-digit ones. She knows the names of complex shapes, including 3D ones. She can apply her knowledge to verbal questions and can demonstrate that she understands addition and multiplication with manipulatives. Her teacher has noticed Amna's eyes shine when she is doing number work at school, and she often asks for maths puzzles in free time.

Concern with justice and fairness

Many children with HLP are concerned with justice and fairness. They may become upset by situations they perceive to be unfair, such as when a rule is applied differently to different people. This can show itself in becoming upset when others around them are treated unfairly, and they can become passionate about human rights issues or animal welfare concerns. It can be an issue in the classroom when certain children are "watched" more closely and sanctions applied unevenly. This can also cause children with high learning potential to question authority about rules they do not understand or do not make sense to them.

Example:

Kai is nine years old and enjoys going to cubs (young boy scouts in the UK). However, he is considering leaving the pack because he finds it difficult to tolerate the leader's attitude towards some of his fellow members. In particular, the leader reprimands Kai's best friend more harshly than Kai when they are equally to blame for a minor misdeed. Kai tried to speak to the leader about it but was met with indifference. The situation is causing him so much distress that it has tainted an activity he loves, and he feels his only choice is to leave the pack.

Sensitivity

This characteristic can apply to both sensory sensitivity and emotional sensitivity. Many children with high learning potential have some sensory processing differences, which is explained in more detail later in this chapter under Dabrowski's Sensual Overexcitability, as well as more extensively throughout the book. It is also common for children with HLP to have exceptional emotional sensitivity; that is to say they experience intense or "big" emotions with others often describing them as "being too sensitive for their own good". Children with HLP's emotional sensitivity and associated behaviours are often due to a sensitivity that they are born with which means they feel things deeply, sometimes due to a fallout of their needs not being met, and sometimes both of these factors. Although their ability to regulate their strong emotions, as seen in their associated behaviour, could be described as expected considering their age, it also often lags behind their peers; and/or especially behind their advanced skills in other areas (see Asynchronous Development later in this chapter). The section on Dabrowski's Emotional Overexcitability explains more about emotional sensitivity, and this is also addressed throughout the book.

Example:

Six-year-old Sky enjoys playing board games with her family, and she can easily understand and play strategy games aimed at nine year olds and above. However, she gets very upset when she is not in the lead or does not win. Frequently, this causes emotional outbursts in which she cries and is inconsolable for up to an hour. She has been known to completely upset the game board when in this state. Her parents have realised that playing games where all the players are trying to win the game together is much better for Sky, but she still gets very upset when the group is losing the game.

Wide range of interests

Having "passions", or topics of intense interest, is common for children with high learning potential, as is having a wide range of interests. This often stems from being interested in how the world around them works and why things happen the way they do. It is frequently linked to being observant and having strong curiosity.

Example:

Benedict is seven years old, and his teacher has noticed he has a lot of intense interests. He is generally interested in maths and science at school but is very interested in robotics and how it is applied in industry and prosthetics, spending time reading and researching these outside of school. Benedict is also interested in politics; he reads a children's weekly newspaper and watches children's news on the TV. He enjoys talking about current affairs and seems to be aware of and understand even more than his teacher about what is going on. In addition, Benedict is interested in football (soccer). He enjoys playing in a team, follows the teams and players in the premier league and understands the statistics behind the leagues, games and players. He has invented a fantasy league and updates his scores weekly in a notebook he keeps.

Profiles of the Gifted and Talented

The Profiles of the Gifted and Talented is a set of profiles that provides a broad set of traits to help identify children with high learning potential. Neihart and Betts first proposed their Profiles of the Gifted and Talented in the journal *Gifted Child Quarterly* in 1988[13] and later revised and refined them in 2010.[14] The Profiles brought together their understanding after years of observations, interviews and reviews of literature and offered parents and professionals an opportunity to consider the feelings, behaviours and needs of the different types of high ability individuals.

Often it is assumed that individuals with high abilities are similar in character to one another, resulting in some, especially those who exhibit traits which do not fit common assumptions, being overlooked and their needs going unmet. The Profiles of the Gifted and Talented tries to bust the myth that we should expect a certain type of character in children identified as having high learning potential, such as being mature or compliant, and encourages parents and professionals to look more widely at how high learning potential presents in children. Indeed, many children with HLP are afraid to take intellectual risks, preferring to stay in their comfort zone, and some are unwilling to show what they are capable of unless they

Table 2.1 Character Traits of Profiles of the Gifted and Talented

Profile	Traits
Successful	Achieves well; good grades; accepts social norms and conforms; absorbs knowledge; avoids risks.
Creative	Perseveres in interests; expresses self creatively; stands up for convictions; honest and direct; questions rules and policies; emotionally labile; poor self-control; impulsive.
Underground	Devalues, discounts or denies talents; rejects academic challenge; unsure of direction; socially unconnected or moves from one group to the next.
At-Risk	Creates disruptions; pursues outside interests; will do academic work when values the relationship with the teacher; inconsistent performance; low attendance; often creative; critical of self and others.
Multi/Twice-Exceptional	Thinks conceptually; good problem-solver; makes connections easily; enjoys novelty and complexity; inconsistent performance; disorganised; slow processing; emotionally dysregulated; may exhibit behaviour problems.
Autonomous	Appropriate social skills; seeks challenge; works independently; strongly self-directed; follows passions; resilient; good understanding and acceptance of self.

really trust the viewer. Table 2.1 summarises the Profiles and their accompanying traits. The Profiles are not meant as a way of categorising individuals but more as a reminder that children with HLP come with a variety of profiles, moving parents and professionals beyond the characteristics and the suggestion that all children with HLP present in the same way.

Successful

Children with HLP who have a Successful Profile are perhaps those who are most easily identifiable since they **tend to fit the typical belief about a child who is ahead for their age, are successful in most situations, can often meet the expectations of adults and conform to social norms**.

This group of children tends to have quite positive self-esteem and is happy to put in effort for the rewards and praise offered by parents or teachers, meaning their motivation is generally extrinsic. This may set them up to fail in future unless they learn to do things for their internal reward. They may well experience boredom because work is not at the right level for them or things do not go quickly enough for them. Children with a Successful Profile are often afraid of taking risks so shy away from experiences that may challenge them and choose "safe" activities instead. Indeed, they may well be of a "fixed" mindset (see Chapter 6 for more about growth/fixed mindset).

For this group of children, to avoid the pitfalls, it is important that they are challenged in their learning so they learn to be okay outside their comfort zone and become comfortable with taking risks. Having the opportunity to develop their creativity through the arts is one of the ways in which they can learn to do this. It is also important for them to learn to understand more about their own thought patterns to be able to understand why they avoid risks and be able to persist through them. In early education, many Successful Profile children will have found learning easy and expect to be able to do the same as they progress through the education system, but this is not always the case when learning material gets more complicated, so developing their study skills is also essential for this group.

Creative

The next group describes the Creative Profile, sometimes called the Challenging Profile, of children with HLP. Children in this group are **highly creative thinkers and are less likely to put in effort for external reward, preferring to be self-driven and follow their own passions.** They often get bored and frustrated since they crave challenges to their thinking and become impatient when their brains are not working. Their self-esteem is high at times and low at others. They may become impatient with others when they do not see things from their perspective or when they do not catch on as quickly as them. They often have heightened emotional sensitivity and may experience meltdowns. As a result of their sensitivity, they may be more psychologically vulnerable, with many from this group suffering from anxiety and depression as they get older. They are often passionate about causes and have that sense of justice and fairness which was mentioned in the characteristics section.

Creative Profile children with HLP are the most likely to **question authority**, since they have the self-esteem and passion to do this. They often question the rules and policies, especially when they see them applied inconsistently. Standing up for their convictions may well contribute to this questioning of authority. Creative Profile children often speak in an honest and direct way, a trait that therapists dealing with them will need to understand and cope with, and that we discuss further in Chapter 6. As mentioned above, their emotional sensitivity means they have poor self-control resulting in outbursts and mood swings, and this may also affect their relationships with their peers.

To support these Creative Profile children, adults around them need to understand that creativity and creative thinking is important for them to have, and they need the opportunity to exercise and develop this. Despite struggles with their peers, they also need to be able to feel connected to others, and so opportunities to develop relationships around their interests is important. Creative Profile children need less pressure to conform, not more, so that they can be happy with who they are rather than feeling like they need to try and dampen their being. Again, with this group, there is a need for them to be aware of who they are, to understand their thought patterns so that they can develop tact, flexibility, self-awareness and control, which will have a knock-on effect on the ability to maintain friendships.

Underground

Children with HLP who have an Underground Profile tend to be more **ambivalent about achievement and feel very unsure about themselves. They have a desire to belong socially but struggle to find where they fit.** They often feel very different to the family or background they come from and so feel conflicted, carry some guilt and are insecure. They are unsure of their right to their emotions and so have an almost diminished sense of self in that they are not sure of their own identity. This results in children from this group being susceptible to peer pressure and experiencing empathy overload.

Children with an Underground Profile tend to **deny their talents** and are unlikely to grab opportunities to develop which present themselves. They resist accessing more challenging levels of education since they suffer from imposter syndrome, feeling as if they don't have a right to be there. Socially, they move from one peer group to the next, never really settling. Nor do they feel part of a class at school. They feel very unsure of their direction in life.

Children with HLP from the Underground group need to have the freedom to make choices and be heard. It is important that children in this group also have the opportunity to be aware of their thought-life to foster their self-understanding and acceptance of themselves. In order to develop their sense of identity, children from this group need support for their abilities and interests.

At-Risk

Children with HLP with an At-Risk Profile tend to suffer from **poor mental health, having a poor self-concept, being resentful and angry, feeling isolated and being prone to depression.** They often experience explosive outbursts, act defensively and are resistant to authority. They may put themselves into risky situations since they have little fear. Their motivation to work is very unlikely to be for grades, but they will put in work once they have built a good relationship with the teacher.

Children within this group are likely to have poor attendance at school and may experience school refusal.[*] They rarely complete a task and seem disengaged from classwork. However, they tend to be creative and will often pursue interests in their own time. They are very critical of both themselves and others. They may self-isolate and/or self-harm.

Since this group of children is at-risk, they need an alternative to the traditional education environment. Indeed, some from this group may already be excluded[†] from mainstream school, attending an alternative[‡] or blended[§] provision, or their parents may be electively home educating them. This is because they need a programme of learning that is tailored to their needs and interests with intensive support. The mental health needs of this group mean that these children will need some form of counselling or therapy. Discussion about their interests, direction and short-term goals would also be helpful to the At-Risk Profile children with HLP.

Multi/Twice-Exceptional

Multi or Twice-Exceptional (also known as DME or 2e) Profile children with HLP are those who **have a special educational need or learning difference, physical disability or mental health need alongside their advanced abilities**. The topic of children with DME/2e is covered in much greater depth in Chapter 3 and throughout the rest of the book. Children with a Multi/Twice-Exceptional Profile tend to suffer from intense frustration and anger, as well as poor self-concept and feelings of inferiority. They have to put in a lot of effort just to get by with everyday life and so struggle to view themselves as successful. They lack confidence and struggle to fit in socially.

This group of children are **very good problem solvers** since their brains can think outside the traditional boxes. They make connections between subjects and topics easily and think conceptually, working from concept to detail rather than the usual other way around. However, in school they may seem to be working at the expected standard for their age or below, and their achievements are likely to be inconsistent depending on whether things are working in their favour on the day of assessment or pieces of work. They are often disorganised and may be disruptive in class.

For this group, it is important to emphasise their strengths and so a strength-based approach tends to support them best. They need support to develop coping and other management skills. Choosing a learning environment that supports them, values their abilities and develops their strengths is important to avoid many pitfalls. This group should be able to access challenging work in their strength areas so they can learn study skills and perseverance in these strength areas. It is also important to be on the lookout for additional, as yet undiagnosed, conditions – especially ADHD.

Autonomous learner

Autonomous Learner Profile children with HLP seem to have it altogether. They are **confident, socially accepted, and willing to fail**. They understand themselves well, which means they can apply this understanding to ensure that conditions are right for them to succeed. They have a desire to know and learn for learning's sake, and they are enthusiastic about learning. They have an intrinsic motivation and seek personal satisfaction. They tend to have support from their parents or others. Since they feel supported and can accept themselves, they are also able to accept others.

This group of children have social skills that mean they can fit in and are rarely bullied. They are able to pursue their interests and academic work independently, developing their own short-term and longer-term goals. They stand up for their convictions and are **resilient in the face of setbacks**.

Even children in this group who have so much going for them have needs that require support. Autonomous learner children with HLP need advocacy since they often do not have a voice themselves, such as to access higher level education activities. These children also need feedback about their strengths and the possibilities for new directions they could take. They need some input to facilitate their personal growth and some support for risk-taking. This could take the form of a mentoring or coaching relationship. This would also support their increased independence as they mature.

HLP profiles summary

The explanation of these profiles should give you a flavour of the different ways that high learning potential can present itself in individual children. Indeed, reading about the profiles may bring to mind children occupational therapists have worked with. All of the children the profiles describe have needs and require support, but the type of support will differ based on their profile. Occupational therapists are in a position to be able to support children with high learning potential who come to them, whatever their profile and needs, but understanding the child and what is going on for them is key to getting the support right. It is most likely that the children occupational therapists come across have some additional learning needs, which means they are dual or multiple exceptional/2e and therefore have elements of the Multi/Twice-exceptional Profile. However, children do not necessarily fit neatly into a profile and so these children could also have elements of one or more of the other profiles. In Chapter 3 and throughout the rest of the book, we discuss children with dual or multiple exceptionality/twice exceptionality and how to consider their individual personalities and needs further.

Asynchronous Development

There is one definition of gifted individuals that voices what many think about the difference of experience of those with high cognitive abilities/achievement. It embodies the neurodiversity-affirming approach to high learning potential and acknowledges that the inner thoughts and experience of the world of gifted people may be different to neurotypical individuals. The definition also introduces the term asynchronous development, which this section is all about. It is called the Columbus Group definition:

> Giftedness is asynchronous development in which advanced cognitive abilities and heightened intensity combine to create inner experiences and awareness that are qualitatively different from the norm. This asynchrony increases with higher intellectual capacity. The uniqueness of the gifted renders them particularly vulnerable and requires modifications in parenting, teaching and counseling in order for them to develop optimally
>
> *(The Columbus Group, 1991).*[15]

The Columbus Group gathered in the early 1990s in Columbus Ohio in the USA, in response to the increasing emphasis on achievement through the "talent development model" in the world of gifted research, which tended to ignore the emotional needs of children with high learning potential. Comprising researchers, educators and psychologists, this group of five women with extensive experience in the field agreed that what was common between the children they worked with was they were out of sync with age-related expectations; they were many ages at the same time. They proposed the term asynchronous development to describe this phenomenon and concluded that it caused the unique emotional needs of this group of children. According to one article written by a member of the group at the time, asynchronous development places gifted individuals outside normal developmental patterns from birth to adulthood.[16]

28 *High Learning Potential (HLP)/Giftedness*

In addition, Dr James Webb, psychology professor and gifted education researcher also stated:

> Gifted children often have substantial variations in abilities within themselves and develop unevenly across various skill areas… because it is prominent in so many gifted children, some professionals believe asynchronous development, rather than potential or ability, is the defining characteristic of giftedness.[17]

Having one or more areas significantly ahead for their years already means a child with high learning potential is developing asynchronously. The higher the cognitive ability, the more different to the norm their experience is likely to be. Asynchronous development means that there are gaps between different areas of a child's development and this can lead to misunderstandings and frustration. One example of asynchronous development is a child whose reading level is four years ahead of their chronological age whilst their handwriting level is at the same level as their peers. This represents a significant gap between the two. Similarly, a child may have maths understanding and skills that are three years ahead for their age, yet struggle with emotional regulation which would be considered immature for their years. There are many more examples, and every child who has high learning potential

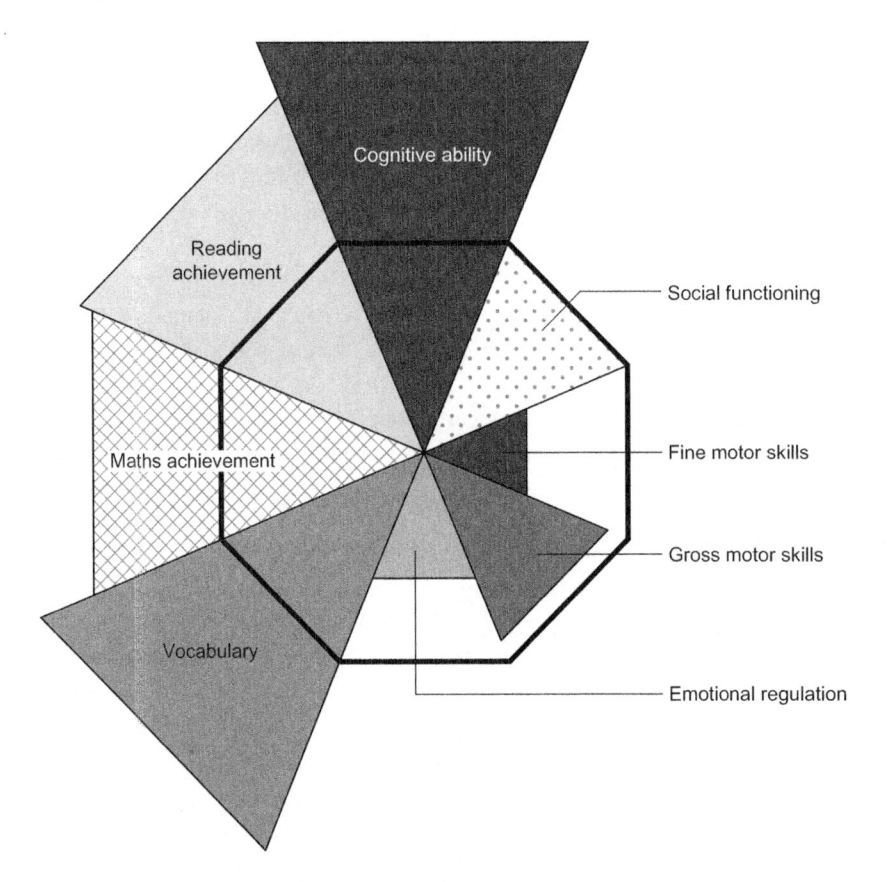

Figure 2.2 Asynchronous development.

will have some form of asynchronous development. In fact, relevant areas of development in an individual could be plotted on a chart similar to that in Figure 2.2 to understand how asynchronous development affects them uniquely.

It is important to understand how asynchronous development may be affecting a child in terms of the misunderstandings and frustration it may cause. For example, a child who has a lot of ideas in their head but does not have the skills to be able to write them down is likely to become frustrated when they are able to talk about a topic eloquently but cannot fulfil their teacher's expectation of being able to put a similar level of language into their writing. The teachers may well misunderstand the reason for the child not showing their language skills through their writing and deliver harmful messages to the child rather than encouraging them appropriately. Another example is that a child who can read at a level several years above their age may struggle to emotionally cope with concepts in books aimed at older children. Adults around the child may jump to the wrong conclusion about why the child is upset and feel it best to restrict their reading material, which could stifle their development, when it would be better to discuss the issue with the child and decide on appropriate support together.

Children who have a special educational need or disability in addition to their high learning potential will have, by definition, at least one area of development that is lagging behind their chronological age in addition to some areas that are advanced. This means that the gaps between areas of development are even wider in this group of children and, therefore, their asynchronous development is likely to lead to even more frustration and misunderstanding.

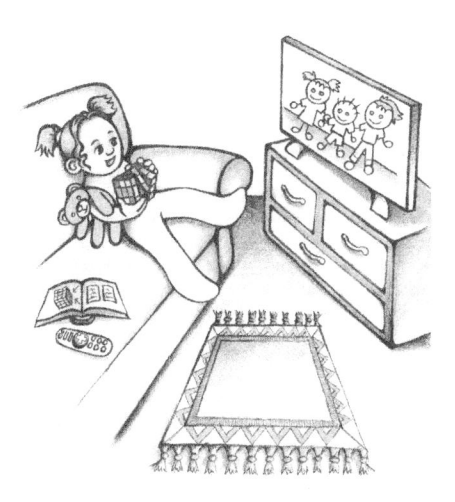

Parents of gifted children sometimes highlight the juxtapositions of their children's asynchronous development, and these real-life quotes from an online support group can highlight the extremes.

Parent quotes about their children's asynchronous development

"Malik – age 5 – was just watching Go Jetters [a TV programme aimed at preschoolers] then almost solved a 5x5 Rubik's cube".

"My 2-year-old has been identifying the pupil and the iris in eyes for a while now. Today she kept saying 'I'm dripping. Crying made me drip!' It took me ages to figure out what she was on about, because it never occurred to me that she didn't know what tears were called"!

"My daughter: 'Everyone either calls me too baby-ish or too old; I'm never the same age as them'".

"My three-year-old just asked me to write 'right' and 'left' in his shoes because, although he can read both those words, and knows which is which, he can't get his shoes on the 'correct feet'".

"Rosanna is average to below average with maths and reading but in speech, vocabulary, language comprehension, knowledge and understanding of the world, comprehension, memory etc. etc. she is light years ahead, far beyond her age. I am a primary school teacher and I know she is operating in those areas around age eight to nine. She just turned six a few weeks ago".

"I've just played chess against my four-year-old (who has complex needs and has never been taught, just been around in the background sometimes while I've been learning to play alongside my six-year-old). She's picked up how the game works just from hovering in the background and kept rambling gameplans of at least 15 to 20 steps the whole time we were playing, but constantly confuses 'pawns' and 'prawns', despite the six-year-old correcting her approximately every three and a half seconds".

"Asynchronous development at its best: our six-year-old making a digestive system (with food going through it) out of Play-Doh. This was after discussing tetragraphs with her dad".

"Liam (age seven) and his toy monkey are watching an exam board video of GCSE biology practicals".

"My three-year-nine-month old is doing an age seven to eight maths workbook (his choice) but still wearing a nappy".

"Asynchronous development: when your child can add multiple amounts within seconds but still reverses the number two".

To further illustrate what asynchronous development means, consider this quote from an article written by Morelock called "Giftedness: The View from Within"[18]:

Consider four-year-old Jennie. Jennie's grandfather died several months ago; Jennie is asking questions about death and showing evidence of emotional upset. Her mother tries to reassure her by telling her that she need not worry. Her mother explains that she and Jennie's father will live for many years. She also explains that Jennie will have her own children and that her mother would become their grandmother to them. Jennie responds to this in trembling voice, 'But you don't know, Mommy. Even children die sometimes. Nobody knows for sure...'

Typical four year olds would just accept reassurance from a parent but Jennie has high learning potential meaning and her reasoning abilities are exceptional for her age. Morelock goes on,

> They create for her a reality more complex and threatening than that facing her age mates. Like average four-year-olds, she needs to believe her mother in order to feel emotionally secure. However, her advanced cognitive capacities allow her to see too clearly the faulty logic. She is left vulnerable and bereft of comfort.

Potential Plus UK, a charity supporting the needs of children with high learning potential, summarises it well, stating that:

> The main reason for high learning potential children's social and emotional vulnerability is asynchronous development, whereby intellectual development is out of sync with social, emotional and/or physical development.[19]

Dr. Linda Silverman, Director of the Institute for Advanced Development and the Gifted Development Center in the USA, hails asynchronous development as "a child-centred perspective that can guide parenting, teaching and counselling of gifted children".[20] She goes on to state that "Giftedness as asynchrony offers both an understanding of the inner experience of gifted individuals throughout the lifespan and a sound framework for responding to the developmental differences of this group". It is clear that having thinking abilities several years above chronological and physical age, in some cases a gap of six or eight years between the two, poses a unique set of challenges for an individual to navigate. The examples above illustrate everyday life with children who have these challenges. As Dr. Silverman suggests, professionals working with children with HLP can respond to these developmental differences in their practice once they are aware of them, and this applies to occupational therapists too.

Dabrowski's Overexcitabilities

Another lens through which we can view high learning potential or giftedness is that of overexcitabilities, which can be seen threaded through the frameworks already considered in this chapter. The term refers to hypersensitivities that many individuals with high learning potential experience, and that have an impact on their lives. Understanding these overexcitabilities helps to explain further the assertion that people with high learning potential experience the world differently since the construct provides a framework for these hypersensitivities. Occupational therapists will see some of the differences that their work addresses reflected in the overexcitabilities, and this is also further discussed in Chapter 5.

Overexcitabilities are part of the Theory of Positive Disintegration (TPD) posited by Kazimierz Dąbrowski, Polish psychologist and psychiatrist (1902-1980). The theory describes a process of personality development, and the creation of a unique, individual personality. It is a complex theory that introduced several new terms and constructs. Unlike mainstream psychology, TPD views psychological tension and anxiety as necessary for personal growth. These "disintegrative" processes are positive in that they lead to growth. Some people possess development potential and so are more likely to experience disintegration and therefore progress through levels of personality development. Many factors are incorporated in developmental potential, but there are three main aspects: overexcitability (OE), specific abilities and talents, and a strong drive toward autonomous growth.

The latter two of these speak for themselves but the overexcitabilities take a little more explanation. Overexcitabilities can be described as **heightened experiences of stimuli that result from increased sensitivities. It is said that the greater the overexcitability, the more intense the individual's experiences of life**. According to Dabrowski, there are five forms of overexcitability: psychomotor, intellectual, emotional, sensual and imaginational. These overexcitabilities often cause a person to profoundly feel the joys and sadness of life and to experience daily life more intensely. See Table 2.2 for a description of each overexcitability.

Table 2.2 Description of Dabrowski's Overexcitabilities

Overexcitability	Description
Psychomotor	**Enhanced excitability of neuromuscular system**
	Characterised by a surplus of energy, rapid speech, busyness and restlessness, intense physical activity, gestures with the whole body, impulsive actions, compulsive talking or activity, a pressure for action, fidgeting and fiddling.
Intellectual	**Intensified activity of the mind**
	Characterised by constant activity of the mind, thought and thinking about thinking, a search for truth, tenacity in problem solving, forming new ideas, intense curiosity, sustained intellectual effort, avid reading and keen observation.
Emotional	**Heightened emotions and exceptional sensitivity**
	Characterised by strong emotional expression, sometimes somatic (both positive and negative, sometimes extreme or complex), identification of others' feelings, capacity for strong emotional attachments and deep relationships, strong emotional memory, inner dialogue and self-judgement, strong empathy, compassion and responsiveness to others.
Sensual	**Sensory aspects of life heightened**
	Characterised by a sensitivity to sensory stimuli, delight in beautiful objects, strong reactions to music, aesthetic interests, a need for sensory comfort, an increased need to touch/be touched, enhanced aesthetic appreciation.
Imaginational	**Capacity to visualise extremely well**
	Characterised by invention and fantasy, detailed visualisation, elaborate and vivid dreams, imaginary worlds and friends, dramatisation, visualising the worst possible outcomes and situations, low tolerance of boredom and a need for variety and novelty.

Dabrowski carried out research with intellectually gifted and artistically talented children in 1967 and found that every one of his 80 subjects had overexcitabilities. He hypothesised that

> as a group the children identified as gifted will tend to display stronger development potential (and overexcitabilities), increased levels of psychoneuroses, and will be predisposed to experience positive disintegration.[21]

The Theory of Positive Disintegration and concept of overexcitabilities were introduced to the world of gifted education by Michael Piechowski in 1979. He went on to develop a questionnaire about overexcitabilities, which was later revised following some criticism. The Overexcitability Questionnaire-Two (OEQ-II) is an instrument to measure overexcitabilities, and its development has aided much research into the concept over the past 40 years, although its validity remains uncertain, and there are many questions unanswered. Unfortunately, other research does not help clarify whether there indeed are psychological differences between children with high learning potential and those who have typical cognitive development. Some studies conclude there are none and others highlight differences, such as the overexcitabilities, being more prevalent, and there being a higher rate of depression and anxiety in the gifted group.

Certainly, children with high learning potential, their parents and educators, not to mention gifted adults, find it helpful to have the overexcitabilities concept to describe their experiences and sensitivities so that they can understand themselves better and use the terms in communicating their experiences to others.

Occupational therapists will likely recognise some or all the overexcitabilities in the children with HLP they work with. Having an increased understanding of the range of overexcitabilities and how it can impact on the daily lives of these children will undoubtedly equip therapists to better help them. Therapists will also be able to make the connection that some of these overexcitabilities are indeed the hypersensitivities they deal with and provide direct therapy for on a daily basis; in particular the psychomotor and sensual overexcitabilities and their overlap with sensory processing differences that we discuss in Chapter 5 in the context of occupational therapy. In fact, therapists will also deal with the other overexcitabilities to support children with HLP's wellbeing and thought patterns. To provide further illustration of how the overexcitabilities can manifest in children with HLP, we have given some examples below.

Example of Psychomotor Overexcitability:

Charlotte is a busy nine year old who is always on the move. Her parents call her a chatterbox who always has something to say. They have realised that the best thing to keep her fulfilled is to feed her constant need to move. So, they have arranged for her to take part in several physical activities each week: gymnastics, swimming, tennis and drama clubs. Charlotte is very animated when she talks, and people tend to gravitate towards her because she is exciting to be around. However, she often interrupts people and gets into trouble at school for talking too much.

Example of Intellectual Overexcitability:

Nate is a five year old who loves to learn and use his mind. He seems to constantly need his mind to be stimulated while he is awake and struggles to get to sleep because his mind is still active. He enjoys finding out information and his current favourite topics are Greek myths, philosophy and artificial intelligence. His mother takes him to the library each week where he maxes out his library card and reads all the books by the following visit. Nate loves having conversations with adults who speak to him just like another adult and who will discuss his favourite topics with him. He also loves to work through logic, word and escape puzzles.

Example of Emotional Overexcitability:

Marilyn is an eight year old who feels all the emotions to a great extent: joy, sadness, anger, fear and anxiety. Marilyn suffers frequent stomach aches. At first her parents thought she was ill and kept her off school, but they have found no medical reasons for the stomach aches and realised they coincide with when she has fallen out with friends at school or when a test is approaching. Her big feelings result in joy expressed physically - often bouncing up and down when she is excited - and in outbursts when she is angry as she is unable to contain herself. Marilyn finds it difficult to watch movies, even Disney movies, because she identifies so strongly with the characters' feelings that she becomes upset when something bad happens to them.

Example of Sensual Overexcitability:

Ten-year-old Daryl is very sensitive to sensory input, especially to noise and touch. He finds it difficult to use public toilets when out and about with his family since the hand dryers make a very big noise. He loves the theatre, especially musical theatre, but he struggles with the loud noises and cracks that happen during a performance. His family has gotten used to this and are sure to ask whether and when such noises might happen during the performances they go to see so that he can cope. Daryl plays several musical instruments, and people enjoy listening to him as he puts so much emotion into the performance. Daryl says his happy place is when he is listening to music through headphones - as he gets "lost" in the music and experiences a sense of euphoria.

Example of Imaginational Overexcitability:

Sammy-Jo is four years old and she is engaged in some sort of role play most of the time. She has invented a world in which she is a witch who creates potions, casts spells and has a menagerie. Each of her animal friends has a name and she often gets her father to play the witch's cat. She creates elaborate scenarios that people around her – siblings, other family members and friends – are asked to take part in. If no one is around to take part, this is not a problem for Sammy-Jo. She just gets one of her many pretend friends to join in. Sammy-Jo often has vivid and complex dreams that she recites in detail to her father when she wakes. Sometimes Sammy-Jo catastrophises about family members dying or the car they are travelling in crashing. She becomes upset and her father finds it difficult to comfort her.

Summary of Needs of Children with High Learning Potential

Having learned about the characteristics, differing profiles, asynchronous development of and the overexcitabilities that children with high learning potential experience, occupational therapists will have an increased understanding of how these children may present and can start to recognise them better when they enter the therapy room or as therapists get to know them. The needs of children with HLP have been touched upon throughout this chapter, but we bring them together here. Their needs also bring about certain risks. We therefore place the needs and risks in the following categories to bring some clarity to the subject.

Hypersensitivity

Children with HLP often have one or more of the hypersensitivities outlined in the section on Dabrowski's overexcitabilities. These kinds of hypersensitivities, especially the psychomotor and sensual ones, are present in children with HLP who have additional learning differences (DME/2e) to an even greater degree. This means their experience of life is different to that of typically developing children, and this needs understanding and accommodation if they are to thrive.

Misunderstanding

Children with HLP are often misunderstood for several reasons: they seem mature in many ways and yet some areas of their development are not at the same level as their advanced abilities and/or their peers (asynchronous development); they seem to want to connect with children the same age but fail to find similar-minded peers; they experience hypersensitivities that alter their life experience and this is not apparent to onlookers. The misunderstanding by and of peers sometimes results in children with HLP being bullied.[22]

Missing out on appropriate education

Children with HLP often have needs that are unrecognised in school settings. They are left doing work that is too low a level for them, learning does not progress quickly enough for them, or they are covering work that they already know. All of which means they are learning very little (or nothing at all). They are not developing study skills and resilience through getting stuck on difficult learning material and working to get past difficult problems. This can result in disengagement from learning, resulting in underachievement.

Perfectionism

Often cited as one of the main features of the social and emotional lives of children with HLP, perfectionism is described as striving to be flawless and often involves being critical of imperfections. Whilst perfectionism can be a driver for children with HLP to perform, and to outperform their own previous attempts, if not kept in check it can cause considerable stress and is linked to depression and anxiety. Perfectionism is thought to occur in children with HLP due to their ability to understand what excellence looks like whilst not yet having developed the skills to be able to perform at that level. Perfectionism can be exacerbated by young children with HLP finding much of early learning easy without really trying. They therefore do not encounter failure very often and fail to develop resilience. As learning progresses, children with HLP encounter more complex concepts and the need to develop skills that take a lot of practice, such as fluent writing. This causes them to become despondent, experience frustration and emotional outbursts and feel that they must be doing something wrong.

Feelings of frustration

Children with HLP often experience feelings of frustration due to the above factors or being misunderstood and missing out on an appropriate education. However, because they are young, the children themselves do not necessarily know this is the reason for their frustration. The frustration causes them stress and this manifests in different ways: dissatisfaction, low self-esteem, school refusal, depression and/or anxiety – to name but a few.

Behavioural issues

The misunderstanding, lack of an appropriate education, hypersensitivities and resulting feelings of frustration could all result in children with HLP attempting to communicate their discontent through their behaviour. This behaviour, whether it is becoming upset, having emotional outbursts, being mean to others, using inappropriate language or becoming violent, is all a form of communication, but it is likely to be considered inappropriate by parents or teachers.

Poor mental health

The factors above, as mentioned, could lead to low self-esteem and frustration. This in turn, after a prolonged period with no resolution or change, could result in poor mental health, particularly in children who do not have a supportive family. It is especially common for children with HLP who have hypersensitivities to experience depression or anxiety.[23]

Conclusion

The information given in this chapter should help occupational therapists understand more about children with high learning potential. Keeping in mind the characteristics, profiles, asynchronous development and overexcitabilities will help therapists to recognise such children in their practice.

The end of the chapter brought together the needs of children with high learning potential, allowing therapists to have an understanding of the needs so they can better support children. Chapter 3 looks more closely at children who fit the dual or multiple exceptional/twice exceptional profile.

Notes

* School refusal is a term used in the UK to describe a regular refusal to attend school or routine problems staying at school. Children may avoid school to cope with stress or fear for a vast number of reasons.
† Exclusion refers to when a child is removed from school temporarily or permanently in the UK. Suspension is also used for temporary exclusions. Expulsion is a term used in other parts of the world to mean the same.
‡ Alternative provision is a term used in the UK to describe a category of schools that support children who cannot access mainstream schools.
§ Blended provision or education describes when a child has a combination of educational provision. The provision is often partially online and partially face-to-face.

References

1. Subotnik, R. F., Olszewski-Kubilius, P., & Worrell, F. C. (2011) *Rethinking giftedness and gifted education: A proposed direction based on psychological science.* Psychological Science in the Public Interest, 12(1), 3–54.
2. Omahen, E. (2021) *Evaluating a Child with Autism.* Autism Parenting Magazine. Retrieved on 15 February 2023 from https://www.autismparentingmagazine.com/evaluating-a-child-with-autism/.
3. Pfeiffer, Steven. (2015). *Tripartite Model of Giftedness and Best Practices in Gifted Assessment.* Revista de Educacion. 155-182. 10.4438/1988-592X-RE-2015-368-293.
4. Department for Education (2019) *Schools, Pupils and their Characteristics: January 2019* www.gov.uk/government/statistics/schools-pupils-and-their-characteristics-january-2019.
5. Sutton Trust, *Potential for success: Fulfilling the promise of highly able students in secondary schools*, July 2018 https://www.suttontrust.com/wp-content/uploads/2019/12/PotentialForSuccess.pdf https://researchbriefings.files.parliament.uk/documents/CBP-9065/CBP-9065.pdf.
6. Department for Children, Schools and Families (2008) *Identifying gifted and talented learners - getting started* https://webarchive.nationalarchives.gov.uk/ukgwa/20080910130301/http:/ygt.dcsf.gov.uk/FileLinks/894_new_guidance.pdf.
7. Silverman, L. K., & Waters, J. L. (1988, November) *The Silverman/Waters Checklist: A new culture-fair identification instrument.* National Association for Gifted Children 35th Annual Convention, Orlando, FL. https://www.spart5.net/cms/lib07/SC01000802/Centricity/Domain/491/Characteristics_Scale.pdf.
8. Vialle, W. (2011) *Giftedness from an Indigenous Perspective.* Australian Association for the Education of the Gifted and Talented. Asia-Pacific Conference on Giftedness (11th: 2010: Sydney, Australia), ISBN 978-0-9808448-1-8.

9. Caropreso, E. J., & White, C. S. (1994). *Analogical Reasoning and Giftedness: A Comparison between Identified Gifted and Nonidentified Children.* The Journal of Educational Research, 87(5), 271-278. http://www.jstor.org/stable/27541930.
10. Kanevsky, L. (2013). Tool Kit for High End Differentiation. Burnaby, BC, Canada: Simon Fraser University. (possibilitiesforlearning.com).
11. Hays, C. (2018), *Curiosity and Gifted Identification: A Mixed Methods Study.* Electronic Theses and Dissertations. 1435. https://digitalcommons.du.edu/etd/1435.
12. Shade, R. (1991). *Verbal Humor in Gifted Students and Students in the General Population: A Comparison of Spontaneous Mirth and Comprehension.* Journal for the Education of the Gifted, 14(2), 134-150. https://doi.org/10.1177/016235329101400203.
13. Betts, G. & Neihart, M. (1988). Profiles of the Gifted and Talented. *Gifted Child Quarterly,* 32, 248-253.
14. Betts, G. T., & Neihart, M. (2010). *Revised profiles of the gifted and talented.* Retrieved from Revised profiles of the Gifted and Talented - Neihart and Betts.pdf.
15. Columbus Group (1991, July). Unpublished transcript of the meeting of the Columbus Group. Columbus, Ohio.
16. Morelock, M. J. (1992) *Giftedness: The View from Within.* Understanding Our Gifted. Vol. 4, No. 3, pp. 1, 11-15.
17. Webb, J. T., Gore, J. L., Amend, E. R. & DeVries, A. R. (2007) *A Parent's Guide to Gifted Children.* Great Potential Press.
18. Morelock, M. J. (1992) *Giftedness: The View from Within.* Understanding Our Gifted. Vol. 4, No. 3, pp. 1, 11-15 https://www.davidsongifted.org/gifted-blog/giftedness-the-view-from-within/.
19. Potential Plus UK (n.d.) *Asynchronous Development.* https://potentialplusuk.org/index.php/characteristics/asynchronous-development/.
20. Silverman, L. K. (1997) *The Construct of Asynchronous Development.* Peabody Journal of Education 72 (3&4), 36-58.
21. Tillier, W. (2022) *Dąbrowski 201: An Introduction to Kazimierz Dąbrowski's Theory of Positive Disintegration.* http://www.positivedisintegration.com/Dabrowski201.pdf.
22. Kidscape, (2015) *Supporting high potential learners so they can flourish at school* https://potentialplusuk.org/wp-content/uploads/2018/10/being_me_-_potential_plus_leaflet.pdf
23. Eren F, Çete AÖ, Avcil S, & Baykara B. (2018) *Emotional and behavioral characteristics of gifted children and their families.* Noro Psikiyatr Ars. 2018;55(2):105-112. doi:10.5152/npa.2017.12731.

Chapter three
Dual or Multiple Exceptionality (DME)/Twice Exceptionality (2e)

Introduction

In Chapter 2 we outlined what high learning potential children are like and touched upon dual or multiple exceptionality (DME) within this. A pioneer in this area who developed our understanding about DME/2e, Dr Susan Baum, described children with DME/2e as having complex layers of abilities and difficulties.[1] This complexity brings significant challenges to individuals who have DME/2e. Dr Nicole A. Tetreault explains in her book *Insight into a Bright Mind: A Neuroscientist's Personal Stories of Unique Thinking* (2021),[2] "In my experience, the path of a 2e person is not the easiest road to travel. Even though I have experienced success, I have had equal experiences of failure, frustration and pain." Tetreault echoes the experiences of many children with DME/2e.

Since most of the high learning potential children that occupational therapists come across in their practice will fit into the DME/2e profile, this chapter goes into more depth about what DME/2e is, how to recognise children with DME/2e, and the common barriers they face. To gain even more insight, we present common situations that children with DME/2e find themselves in and the kinds of support these children need. Additionally, we highlight how people with DME/2e are portrayed in the media.

What Is Dual or Multiple Exceptionality (DME) and Twice Exceptionality (2e)?

As discussed in the previous chapter, children with dual or multiple exceptionality (DME) are those who demonstrate exceptional abilities, or potential in one or more areas, while also experiencing challenges or disabilities in another area. This is the term used in the UK to describe children who have both high learning potential and a special educational need or disability (SEND).* It means the same thing as the term twice exceptional, or 2e, which is used in the USA, Australia and various other parts of the world.

Professor Diane Montgomery, one of the UK's foremost writers about the topic, states that dual or multiple exceptionality (DME) is a term "used to describe those who are intellectually very able (gifted) or who have a talent (a special gift in a performance or skill area) and in addition to this, have a special educational need or disability (SEND)".[3]

The term dual or multiple exceptionality reflects the fact that an individual may have more than one issue alongside their high learning potential or giftedness. For example, a person

DOI: 10.4324/9781003334033-3

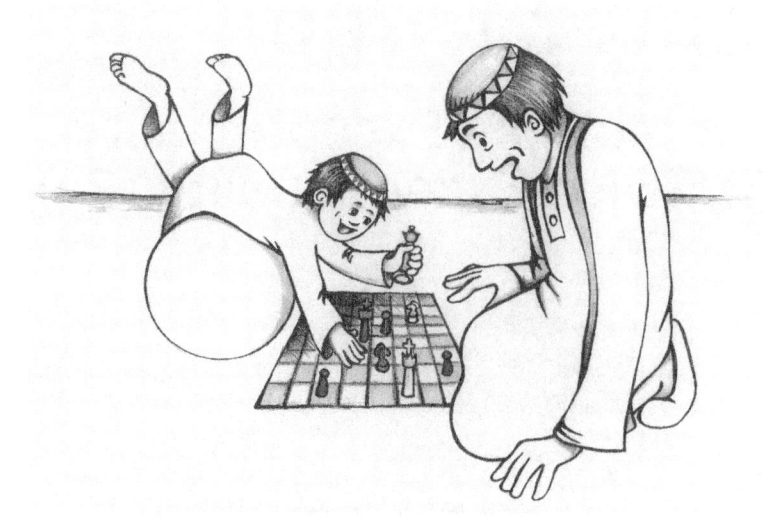

may be autistic and have attention deficit hyperactivity disorder alongside exceptional cognitive abilities. The term first appeared in a government document in 2007[4] that was produced as part of England's national strategy for gifted and talented children in education.

Also discussed in the previous chapter was asynchronous development in reference to children with high learning potential. For children with DME/2e, their asynchronous development presents even wider gaps between different areas of development or achievement. The combination of strengths and weaknesses that children with DME/2e experience can make it difficult for them to navigate academic and social environments, as they are unlikely to fit neatly into traditional categories of "gifted" or "special educational needs". Children with DME/2e are often overlooked or misidentified because their strengths and weaknesses can mask each other.

Examples of children with DME/2e and asynchronous development

Thea:

Thea has very advanced vocabulary and understanding and also has dyslexia. She is able to mask her weaknesses in processing speed and memory and therefore achieves as expected for her age despite having the potential to do much better. The adults supporting Thea do not suspect that she has advanced cognitive abilities, nor that there is an underlying special educational need that is preventing her achieving much more highly.

Olly:

Olly has a visual impairment, advanced reasoning and can carry out advanced mathematical calculations in his head. Olly is held back in his learning and development because he is not given access to materials that would challenge him. Although he is known for being able to give quick answers to sums and being good at problem solving, due to not being able to demonstrate his abilities fully, no one has quite grasped what Olly is capable of.

Emily Kircher-Morris in her book, *Raising Twice-Exceptional Children*, states that "The intersectionality of cognitive ability, neurodivergence, personality, and environmental influences creates a combination of traits that makes each twice-exceptional person completely unique".[5] To understand the range of advanced abilities and special educational needs and disabilities that could make up a child with DME's profile, Ronksley-Pavia's Model of Twice Exceptionality[6] is shown in Figure 3.1.

The model shows two intersecting circles showing areas of giftedness on the right and areas of disability on the left. Where any of the two intersect, Ronksley-Pavia states that this would be a twice exceptional, or DME, profile. The areas of giftedness listed are based

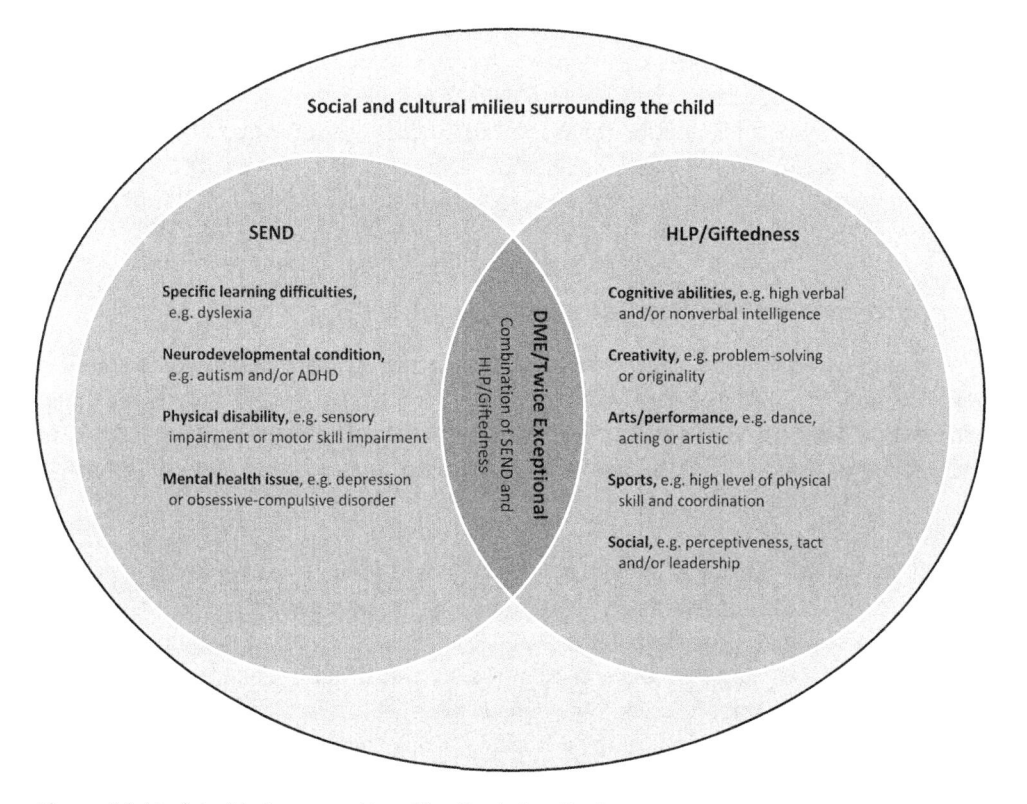

Figure 3.1 Model of twice exceptionality, Ronksley-Pavia.

42 DME/Twice Exceptionality (2e)

on the work of Françoys Gagné's Differentiated Model of Giftedness and Talent, published in 2012,[7] and include intellectual, creative, social, perceptual and physical giftedness. The areas of disability are based on the medical model of categorising disability. The list is not exhaustive and it includes specific learning difficulties such as dyslexia, mental illness such as depression, physical disability such as hearing impairments and neurodevelopmental disorders such as autism and ADHD.

How Many Children with DME/2e Are There?

Estimating the number of children with DME/2e in the population is challenging because identifying this profile in children often requires comprehensive testing and evaluation, which may not be available to all children.

Research suggests that the number of children with DME/2e may be higher than previously thought. For the purposes of calculating numbers of children with DME/2e in the UK, we have used a figure of 10% of children who have high learning potential, which means that approximately 156,000 children will have dual or multiple exceptionalities (DME) or twice exceptionality (2e). It is estimated that between 60,000 and 100,000 children in schools (children of school age and in state schools) have DME, the former figure being the estimate from nasen[†] for England alone[8] and the latter being 10% of the estimated number of children with high learning potential in the UK. Children who are diagnosed with DME/2e are not evenly distributed across different populations and communities. For example, some studies have found that children with DME/2e are more likely to come from families with higher socioeconomic status, suggesting that access to resources and educational opportunities may play a role in identification. This means that children with DME/2e from families with lower socioeconomic statuses are likely to be missing out on identification of the facets of their profiles as well as access to appropriate support and education.

How to Recognise Children with DME/2e

Identifying children with DME/2e can be a challenging task, as their high learning potential may mask their special educational need or disability (SEND), or their SEND may mask their high learning potential. However, it is important for occupational therapists to be aware of how to identify children with DME/2e so they can receive appropriate support and interventions to help them thrive.

One of the ways to recognise a child with DME/2e is through their "spiky" profile. This means that a child has considerable strengths in some areas and considerable weaknesses in others. For example, when a child with DME/2e is assessed by an educational psychologist, it would be expected that percentile figures in some areas of cognitive testing were in the high "above average" range to the "upper extreme" or "superior" range and other areas in the average or below average ranges. When plotted on a chart, this would show scores looking "spiky". Some organisations such as the Belin-Blank Center in the USA use the bell curve to plot different areas of development.

DME/Twice Exceptionality (2e) 43

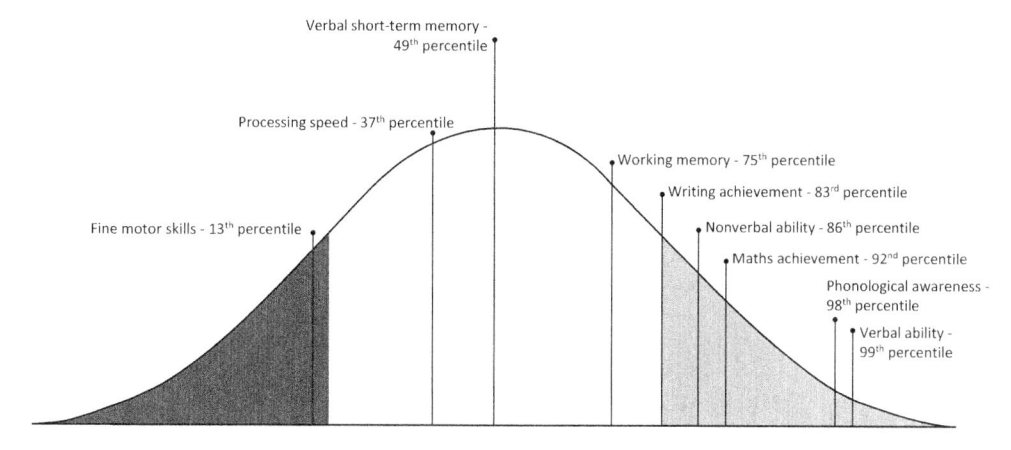

Figure 3.2 Bell curve of development for a child with DME/2e.

Labels on the curve:
- Verbal short-term memory - 49th percentile
- Processing speed - 37th percentile
- Fine motor skills - 13th percentile
- Working memory - 75th percentile
- Writing achievement - 83rd percentile
- Nonverbal ability - 86th percentile
- Maths achievement - 92nd percentile
- Phonological awareness - 98th percentile
- Verbal ability - 99th percentile

A typically developing child would usually have all of the scores for different areas of development plotted within the white, or average, range on the bell normal distribution bell curve. A child with SEND would usually have some of their areas of development (the ones they struggle with) in the dark grey, or below average, range and the rest within the average. However, a child with DME/2e would usually have scores plotted in the light grey, or above average, range as well as the white and dark grey areas. The bell curve of development in Figure 3.2 shows the different areas of development for Teri, an autistic child with high learning potential and motor coordination difficulties. Teri's verbal cognitive ability is on the 99th percentile for their age, indicating that they are performing better than 99% of children their age. Meanwhile, their nonverbal cognitive ability is on the 86th percentile, which is above average for their age but nowhere near their verbal cognitive ability. In itself, this gap highlights that it is likely the child has some neurodiversity. Their phonological awareness is also high, on the 98th percentile. Teri's achievement in reading and maths is close to their cognitive abilities, on the 98th and 92nd percentiles. Due to the motor coordination and social understanding challenges that Teri has, their writing achievement is somewhat lower, on the 83rd percentile, at the top of the "average" range. Teri's working memory can be seen in the "average range", on the 75th percentile, along with their verbal short-term memory which is on the 49th percentile. Teri's processing speed is lower, in the "average" range, on the 37th percentile. Significantly weaker are their fine motor skills, these being on the 13th percentile, in the "below average" range. This is the kind of profile that is described as "spiky"; it shows scores for different areas of development spread across the chart, whatever kind of chart they are plotted on.

With such a profile, the child experiences frustration due to the difference between the higher areas and the lower. The child's high cognitive abilities mean they are able to perceive what good performance is, and they are easily able to compare their performance to that of peers. The high cognitive ability also means the child is able to learn without issue in some areas, in this case reading and maths, yet struggles with other areas of development where their weaknesses affect them more. The child is likely to become very frustrated that they cannot always perform as well as their peers, since they have experienced being successful and do not understand the barriers in their areas of weakness. Additionally, adults around the child may have the expectation that the child will perform well in most things because they have seen them do well in some. This expectation is perceived by the child, and so they experience feelings of confusion, shame and that they have disappointed their parents and educators.

An initial discussion of common characteristics

Whilst it is difficult to generalise about such a diverse group of children, and much will depend on the type of issues experienced alongside their high learning potential, we attempt to firstly discuss the characteristics that children with DME/2e share in brief.

Advanced cognitive ability

As discussed previously, one of the most obvious signs of giftedness is advanced cognitive ability. This includes high levels of intellectual curiosity, creativity, problem-solving skills and abstract reasoning ability. Children with DME/2e are no different in this regard and will certainly have "flashes of brilliance", though they may also have learning impairments or challenges in some areas, as outlined below.

Areas of difficulty

The definition of DME/2e requires that there is a special educational need or disability present in addition to the areas of advanced cognitive ability, whether that SEND is diagnosed or undiagnosed. The areas of weakness in an individual may be due to a condition such as dyslexia, ADHD, autism, or sensory processing differences, because of a disability such as complex physical needs or sensory impairments, or due to mental health problems. The areas of weakness in an individual can contribute or lead to challenges with academic areas such as reading, writing or maths, executive functioning including organisational skills and emotional regulation, attention, social skills or sensory processing.

Uneven development

As mentioned previously, the profile of a child with DME/2e is likely to result in uneven, or asynchronous, development, where their abilities in different areas are significantly higher or lower than their peers. This is one of the tell-tale signs of a child with DME/2e, and results in a whole lot of frustration for them.

Social and emotional challenges

Children with DME/2e may struggle with social skills or emotional regulation, which can make it difficult to form friendships, navigate social situations or regulate their behaviour at home or in the classroom. This also makes it difficult for them to advocate for themselves, and they may become seen as the "naughty" child or the class clown. They may also experience anxiety, depression or other mental health challenges, which is related to their unique needs, experiences and asynchronous development. The challenges and needs that children with DME/2e have may result in behavioural issues when their needs are not met. This may present as impulsivity, hyperactivity, emotional sensitivity or social isolation. These issues may be related to needs caused by their SEND, their giftedness or a combination of both.

Perfectionism

This characteristic was discussed in Chapter 2 in relation to children with HLP. However, mentioning it here again in relation to children with DME/2e is beneficial to draw attention to how it can affect them. Perfectionism can be a sign of both their giftedness and their SEND because they have high expectations of themselves and become frustrated when they are unable to meet them. Children with DME/2e may also feel pressure to excel academically or to hide their learning differences from peers and teachers. Their strong emotions and struggles with emotional or self-regulation may also mean that they struggle to cope with these feelings, resulting in emotional outbursts. Perfectionism can also lead to a cycle of perfectionism, self-doubt and anxiety that can be difficult to break.

Disengagement

A child with DME/2e may become disengaged from school or other activities if they are not challenged or supported appropriately. They may also become bored or frustrated if they are not able to keep up with their peers or are not given opportunities to explore their interests. Particularly following the coronavirus pandemic, there has been an increase in school refusal in England.[9] It is likely that a significant proportion of children experiencing disengagement and school refusal have a DME/2e profile of needs, and schools are not in a position to cater for these specific needs which often require a tailored approach.

Strengths and needs

Research has been carried out to look at the strengths and needs of children with DME/2e in order to support professionals to better understand the profile of this group. Following their work on the subject, Higgins and Nielsen proposed an overview showing common strengths and needs of children with DME/2e.[10] This can be seen in Table 3.1 which provides an overview from their research.

In its Dual or Multiple Exceptionality Fact Sheet,[11] Potential Plus UK categorises the characteristics of children with DME/2e into the four separate areas of intellectual strengths, academic difficulties, emotional indicators and behavioural indicators. These are shown in Figure 3.3.

It is highly likely that a child with DME/2e will have characteristics that fit into all four of the above boxes, although an individual child would be unlikely to exhibit all of the characteristics shown above.

Table 3.1 Strengths and Needs of Children with DME/2e, adapted from Higgins and Nielsen

Strengths	Needs
• Superior vocabulary • Advanced ideas and opinions • High levels of creativity and problem-solving ability • Extremely curious, imaginative and inquisitive • Wide range of interests not related to school • Penetrating insight into complex issues • Specific talent or consuming interest area • Sophisticated sense of humour	• Difficulty with neurotypical social skills • High sensitivity to criticism • Lack of organisational and study skills • Discrepant verbal and performance skills • Poor performance in one or more academic areas • Difficulty with written expression • Stubborn, opinionated demeanour • High impulsivity

Figure 3.3 Characteristics of children with DME/2e. Potential Plus UK.

Intellectual Strengths

- Ability/expertise in one specific area
- Active imagination
- Extensive vocabulary
- Exceptional comprehension
- Excelling at tasks requiring abstract thinking and problem solving
- Excellent visual memory
- Creativity outside school

Academic Difficulties

- Poor handwriting
- Poor spelling
- Difficulty with phonics
- Inability to do simple tasks but ability to do more complex ones
- Success in either maths or language subjects but challenges in the other
- Poor performance under pressure
- Difficulty completing tasks with a sequence of steps but ability to take part in broad-ranging discussions
- Inattentive at times

Emotional Indicators

- Minor failures that create feeling of major inadequacy
- Unrealistically high or low self-expectations
- Feelings of academic ineptitude
- Confusion about abilities
- Strong fear of failure
- Sensitivity to criticism
- Experiences of intense frustration
- Low self-esteem
- Feelings of being different from others
- Difficulty with neurotypical social skills

Behavioural Indicators

- Disruptive in class
- Often off-task
- Disorganised
- Unmotivated
- Impulsive
- Creative when making excuses to avoid difficult tasks
- Can be aggressive at times
- Withdrawn at times

The first box, Intellectual Strengths, outlines the kinds of cognitive abilities that are often seen in children with DME/2e. It is more likely that children with DME/2e have ability and/or expertise in one or a narrow set of areas. This is because they may have impairments that mean certain areas are more difficult for them to access and/or because their passion for the areas of ability or expertise helps them to push through their challenges. The trait of excelling at tasks that require abstract thinking and problem solving is often present due to the exceptional comprehension and alternative-thinking individuals with DME/2e may have. Many children with DME/2e are highly creative, finding a way to express themselves through the creative arts and/or thinking creatively. Some children with DME/2e have excellent visual memories due to the differences in the way their brains work. For some, this translates into an active imagination. Many also have an exceptional vocabulary. Readers will note that some of these relate directly to the overexcitabilities, in particular the intellectual and imaginational overexcitabilities.

In the second box, Academic Difficulties, some of the areas children with DME/2e find challenging in school are set out. Which areas they struggle with will very much depend on what their special educational need or disability is. Some of the items relate to challenges that are part of specific learning difficulties such as dyslexia, dyscalculia or dysgraphia and some relate to more general traits that are common between neurodevelopmental disorders such as autism and ADHD. For example, many children with neurodevelopmental disorders struggle with executive functioning and sensory processing, and these cause children's organisational and activity participation skills to be impaired. There are yet other Academic Difficulties traits that are not listed here which relate to other SENDs, such as sensory or physical impairments, that would also impact on academic skills. What can be noted is that the Academic Difficulties often cause the attainment of children with DME/2e to be uneven; at times they can perform exceptionally well in school and at others they underperform.

In the third box, Emotional Indicators, some of the factors that are in the thought-life of children with DME/2e are laid out. These include the low self-esteem that is often a trait in children with special educational needs, and certainly is the case for children with DME/2e due to their ability to conceive what "excellence" looks like from a mature viewpoint. This can result in feelings of academic ineptitude and/or confusion about their abilities. As mentioned above, a strong fear of failure, or perfectionism, is often present and may include unrealistically high or low self-expectations. This group of children with DME/2e have emotional regulation difficulties and have not yet developed their self-awareness and ability to appropriately self-regulate. These children often present with sensitivity to criticism, intense frustration and minor failures that create feelings of major inadequacy. Many children with DME/2e feel different to their peers and some have difficulty with neurotypical social skills due to the challenges of their special educational needs or disabilities.

The fourth box, Behavioural Indicators, displays some of the ways challenges children with DME/2e manifest, especially when their needs are not being met or accommodated. These behaviours are presented from the viewpoint of an onlooker with a negative perspective. It can be argued that the language used is problematic, but the list of mentioned behaviours

SUPPORT MATERIAL

Figure 3.4 Characteristics of Children with DME/2e Form, designed by M. Ferreira, R. Howell based on characteristics of children with DME/2e.

Name of Child:_____ **Age:**_____
Intellectual Strengths (e.g. ability/expertise in one specific area, active imagination, extensive vocabulary, exceptional comprehension, excelling at tasks requiring abstract thinking and problem solving, excellent visual memory, creativity outside school)
Academic Difficulties (e.g. poor handwriting, poor spelling, difficulty with phonics, inability to do simple tasks but ability to do more complex ones, success in either maths or language subjects but challenges in the other, poor performance under pressure, difficulty completing tasks with a sequence of steps but ability to take part in broad-ranging discussions, inattentive at times)
Emotional Indicators (e.g. minor failures that create feeling of major inadequacy, unrealistically high or low self-expectations, feelings of academic ineptitude, confusion about abilities, strong fear of failure, sensitivity to criticism, experiences of intense frustration, low self-esteem, feelings of being different from others, difficulty with neurotypical social skills)
Behavioural Indicators (e.g. disruptive in class, often off-task, disorganised, unmotivated, impulsive, creative when making excuses to avoid difficult tasks, can be aggressive at times, withdrawn at times)

Copyright material from Mariza Ferreira and Rebecca Howell (2024),
Occupational Therapy for Children with DME or Twice Exceptionality, Routledge

is meant as an identification tool for educators who may use similar terminology. Problems with sensory processing and focussing attention may result in the child often being off-task and/or disruptive in class. Executive functioning difficulties may result in the child being impulsive and/or disorganised. Furthermore, emotional regulation difficulties may result in the child being unmotivated, making creative excuses for avoiding difficult tasks or being aggressive and/or withdrawn at times.

The characteristics can be used as a reflection tool for professionals to think about whether a child is exhibiting a profile of DME/2e. As mentioned previously, a child with DME/2e will usually have some characteristics in each of the four boxes. In Figure 3.4, a form is provided that occupational therapists can use as a prompt to help them consider how the four areas relate to individual children they assess.

Figure 3.5 shows an example of the Characteristics of Children with DME/2e Form completed for a child who has high learning potential, dyslexia and ADHD.

Areas of Difficulty in Children with DME/2e

Children with DME/2e can have a variety of different special educational needs and disabilities alongside their high learning potential, and we discuss this in more depth in Chapters 4 and 5, specifically in relation to the role of the occupational therapist. However, it is good for therapists to know that children with DME/2e also often struggle in the following areas (depending on their profile):

- Executive functioning
- Processing speed
- Working memory
- Study skills

Executive functioning

Executive functions are the cognitive processes that allow us to plan, organise, initiate and monitor our behaviour.[12] Children with DME/2e often struggle with these skills, which can affect their academic performance and participation in daily activities. The development of emotional regulation skills includes an awareness of self and self-monitoring skills, among other areas, and so is inextricably connected to executive functioning.[13] Therapists can provide strategies and interventions to help the child improve their executive functions, such as breaking tasks into smaller steps and using visual aids to help the child develop increased self-awareness of their emotional regulation state.

Processing speed

Processing speed is a cognitive ability and is defined as the time it takes a person to do a mental task or the speed at which an individual can understand and react to the information they receive, whether it be visual (letters and numbers), auditory (language) or movement. In other words, processing speed is the time between receiving a piece of information and

50 *DME/Twice Exceptionality (2e)*

Figure 3.5 Worked example of Characteristics of Children with DME/2e Form.

Name of Child: Heather Maddison	**Age:** 9 years and 5 months

Intellectual Strengths *(e.g. ability/expertise in one specific area, active imagination, extensive vocabulary, exceptional comprehension, excelling at tasks requiring abstract thinking and problem solving, excellent visual memory, creativity outside school)*

Advanced abilities in art; very detailed drawings. Frequently makes up characters and designs magazines. Thinks very creatively; good at problem solving. Remembers things very well when shown visually, e.g. maths problems are worked through with manipulatives or illustrations.

Academic Difficulties *(e.g. poor handwriting, poor spelling, difficulty with phonics, inability to do simple tasks but ability to do more complex ones, success in either maths or language subjects but challenges in the other, poor performance under pressure, difficulty completing tasks with a sequence of steps but ability to take part in broad-ranging discussions, inattentive at times)*

Struggles with spelling. Difficulty with comprehension in longer texts (but not in short paragraphs or bullet-points). Difficulty remembering a series of instructions; needs them provided one by one. Gets distracted easily.

Emotional Indicators *(e.g. minor failures that create feeling of major inadequacy, unrealistically high or low self-expectations, feelings of academic ineptitude, confusion about abilities, strong fear of failure, sensitivity to criticism, experiences of intense frustration, low self-esteem, feelings of being different from others, difficulty with neurotypical social skills)*

Very sensitive to criticism. Gets easily upset. Low self-esteem; confused about some things being easy for them and others being hard when other children find them easy. Strong fear of failure/perfectionism.

Behavioural Indicators *(e.g. disruptive in class, often off-task, disorganised, unmotivated, impulsive, creative when making excuses to avoid difficult tasks, can be aggressive at times, withdrawn at times)*

Often off-task. Difficulty with personal organisation; often forgets and loses things and struggles to keep spaces tidy. Acts impulsively. Has outbursts when frustrated. Feels a keen sense of rejection in relationships.

responding to it. Processing speed is not related to intelligence, meaning that one does not necessarily predict the other, and indeed many children with DME/2e have slow processing speed, especially when compared to their other cognitive abilities.[14] Having a slow processing speed means that some tasks will be more difficult than others, like reading, performing calculations, holding conversations or listening and taking notes. It may also interfere with the executive functions described above because a child who has slow processing speed will have a harder time planning, setting goals, starting tasks, making decisions and paying attention.

Working memory

Working memory is part of executive functioning skills. Working memory is the process that happens when we are asked to hold some information in our brains for a short period while we are doing something else. It is often thought of as a post-it note in the brain. We use our working memory when we are asked to do mental calculations that have more than one step or when we are asked to follow a series of instructions. Children with DME/2e may have impaired working memory for their age, or this cognitive function may be significantly lower than their other cognitive abilities.

Study skills

The problems that children with DME/2e have with executive functions, working memory and processing speed have a significant impact on their study skills. In addition, there is an emotional element at work that means these children struggle to develop appropriate study skills. Firstly, when they are young, many things come easily to them. So much so that they do not have to put in much effort to be successful. As academic learning becomes more complex, study skills are needed, and yet these have not been developed at a younger age. In addition, there may be challenges with executive functioning, including emotional regulation, working memory and/or processing speed. This means that children with DME/2e may need support to work through the emotional elements preventing them from developing such skills and explicit teaching of the most effective ways to learn and tackle homework.

Barriers that Children with DME/2e Face

Not only are children with DME/2e difficult to identify, they often encounter barriers to receiving the support they need. This section outlines some of the common barriers children with DME/2e face to their needs being met.

Despite the many talents and abilities of children with dual or multiple exceptionality, they face unique challenges that can make it difficult for them to reach their full potential. These challenges often stem from the intersection of their giftedness and their learning or developmental differences, which can create a mismatch between their abilities and the expectations placed on them. Below are some of the common barriers that children with DME/2e face:

- Misunderstanding and misidentification
- Inconsistent or inappropriate support

- Limited access to resources
- Stigma and stereotyping

Misunderstanding and misidentification

As discussed in the previous section, identifying children with DME/2e can be challenging, and some may never be properly identified or receive recognition of their strengths and needs. As children with DME/2e's strengths can conceal a learning difficulty, it makes it difficult to identify their special educational need or disability. Even where DME/2e is identified, emphasis can often be placed on supporting SEND to the exclusion of the child's strengths and passions. Additionally, despite a diagnosed learning difficulty, children may achieve as expected for their age or above and so do not qualify for additional support such as through an Education Health Care Plan (EHCP).

A recent DME Trust report on the state of provision for DME children in the UK highlighted this:

> While some learners with DME are identified and/or supported, many remain unidentified and/or unsupported by the education system. A lack of identification or appropriate support has devastating consequences for children with DME, many of whom disengage from learning and suffer with mental health issues, and some of whom are squeezed out of the system in the form of school refusal, exclusion and elective home education.[15]

Inconsistent or inappropriate support

Even when children with DME/2e are identified, they may not receive the support they need to thrive. The typical measures to support a special educational need or disability may not be successful for a child who also has high learning potential since it does not support their learning style or provide the cognitive challenge needed. This is also true for traditional occupational therapy; hence the reason for this book!

Conversely, traditional support for high learning potential children may not be suitable as it is reliant upon basic skills, such as fluent handwriting or following multiple instructions, being in place and dependent on their consistent academic achievement. However, it does not provide the accommodations and individualised tuition necessary for that achievement. As identified in the DME Trust report, general SEND or specific disability-related professional development and training activities for educators and health professionals do not empower them to meet the needs of young people with DME/2e adequately since these do not consider the differing profiles of children with DME/2e.

Limited access to resources

Children with DME/2e and their families may struggle to find resources and support that address their unique needs. This can include access to specialised tutoring or therapy, advocacy and legal support, or educational materials that are tailored to their learning styles and interests. Many parents do find support online via websites and support groups but struggle to find specialists to support their children via the traditional channels.

This book and the training courses we have run hope to address the gap in provision for occupational therapists at least. The aforementioned DME Trust report highlighted that accessing relevant specialists who have expertise in DME/2e is a very important part of the provision for children with DME/2e, with one parent asserting that since starting therapy provided by an occupational therapist with an understanding of DME/2e, "Sensory OT has been life changing for her".

The inconsistency of access to appropriate support carries a financial burden for parents who often end up paying for assessments, educational activities and therapy themselves where it is available.

Stigma and stereotyping

There is often a societal expectation that children with HLP should be high-achieving and "easy" learners, while children with special educational needs and disabilities are seen as less capable or less intelligent. This can lead to stereotypes and stigmatisation of children with DME/2e who do not fit neatly into either category and may face incorrect assumptions or biases from teachers, peers or even their own families. Indeed, as highlighted by Falck in her book *Extreme Intelligence: Development, Predicaments, Implications* (2020),[16] there may be constraints to children with DME/2e being able to show what they are capable of, either because of lack of opportunity or "stereotype threat", i.e. their performance is undermined due to being negatively stereotyped as being academically unsuccessful.

The barriers that children with DME/2e and their families encounter make it difficult for children with DME/2e to thrive academically, socially and emotionally.

Scenarios of Children with DME/2e

Potential Plus UK[17] identifies four different scenarios that children with DME/2e find themselves in. Occupational therapists who suspect a child might have a DME/2e profile can use these scenarios to understand the situation a child might be in and therefore how they are perceived, what expectations are placed on them, the support they may be receiving and how these affect the child. The situations are:

1. HLP is recognised but SEND are unrecognised
2. SEND are recognised but HLP is unrecognised
3. Both HLP and SEND are unrecognised
4. Both HLP and SEND are recognised

HLP recognised but SEND unrecognised

In this scenario, children with DME/2e are perceived as having advanced abilities, yet they are struggling in some areas. Children in this situation are likely to compensate for their

SEND through the use of their advanced abilities, leading to their difficulties being hidden. However, as they get older, the discrepancy between their expected and actual performance widens. These children give the impression of being precocious yet this is contradicted by poor handwriting, forgetfulness or disorganisation, and they may be perceived as not trying hard enough. Indeed, diagnosis of any SEND may happen much later for this group than is usual. It is also possible that a child has their SEND only partially recognised, for example if they have dyslexia and ADHD but only the dyslexia has been diagnosed.

SEND recognised but HLP unrecognised

In the second scenario, children with DME/2e are often noticed for what they cannot do rather than what they can. It is likely that their SEND affects their performance to a greater extent and consequently their advanced abilities are not recognised. Because of this, they are unlikely to be offered extended learning opportunities that cater for or bring out their abilities. They are likely to be underperforming and therefore suffer from low self-esteem. This may result in negative or disruptive behaviours, especially in a school setting. They may, however, be more comfortable showing their talents at home where there is little pressure or perceived limitations.

Both HLP and SEND unrecognised

In the third scenario, the high ability of children with DME/2e masks their SEND and vice versa. They are likely to be performing at an average level or "coasting". Their talents may only surface when they "unlock" due to an opportunity in their strength area. According to Potential Plus UK, this group is most at risk of underachievement, and many only discover the cause of their difficulties in their late teenage years or adulthood.

Both HLP and SEND recognised

In the final scenario, and by far the best one for children with DME/2e to find themselves in, children are more likely to be understood and supported. Due to receiving better support for both their strengths and difficulties, they are more confident advocating for themselves and make adults around them aware of difficulties they are facing. The support this group receives means they are much more likely to be academically challenged and have the opportunities to use their talents and creativity, since they have the support they need to overcome their difficulties. This group is most likely to thrive, avoid mental health issues and develop coping skills. This is why understanding a child with DME/2e's full profile is necessary.

Support That Children with DME/2e Need

Children with DME/2e need a unique set of support and accommodations to help them reach their full potential. In this section, we discuss the support that children with DME/2e need to succeed.

Individualised support

One of the most important things that children with DME/2e need is individualised support. Each child has their own set of strengths and challenges, and their support should be tailored to their specific needs. Wormald, Rogers and Vialle (2015)[18] state, "The resources, both physical, psychological, academic, and medical, not to mention the personnel involved, directly affect the multi-exceptional child's academic achievement as much as the child's own capacity and disability do". Individualised support should comprise the strength-based approach of providing academic challenge in strength areas, accommodations for academic challenges, understanding and adaptations for the child's cognitive style, the development of positive relationships and promoting the child's development of their understanding of themselves and how they can learn best. One-to-one support or therapy for certain parts of their functional and cognitive challenges would certainly contribute positively to their overall support. The package of support needed can sometimes be achieved through the use of an Education Health Care Plan (EHCP), which outlines and provides for the accommodations and modifications the child needs to thrive. In the context of occupational therapy, this is one of the reasons why we feel the DME-C therapy approach is best provided on a one-to-one basis for a child, as opposed to being provided in group format.

Understanding and empathy

As mentioned in the previous chapter, children with DME/2e often feel misunderstood and frustrated by their own limitations. It is important for parents, educators and therapists dealing with children with DME/2e to gain an understanding of the unique challenges they face. This understanding can help to build empathy and create a supportive environment. As Hirt says in her book *Boost: 12 Effective Ways to Lift Up Our Twice-Exceptional Children* (2018),[19] "I realised I needed to give up my preconceived ideas of what parenting was supposed to be; I was determined to start fresh once I was armed with my new understanding. This is important for educators as well". Adults around children with DME/2e should also be aware of the social and emotional challenges that these children may face and support them to develop self-awareness and self-understanding. Providing a safe and supportive environment can help children with DME/2e to feel more comfortable and confident in their abilities.

Appropriate academic challenges

Children with DME/2e require appropriate challenges in their educational setting. They need to be challenged academically, but also need support when they struggle with certain tasks. This balance of challenge and support is crucial in ensuring their needs are met. In particular, it is important to adopt a strength-based approach for children with DME/2e. They will certainly benefit from opportunities to pursue their interests and passions since they are more likely to push past struggles and develop study skills when working in these areas. Developing their interests and passions will also help children with DME/2e to build their confidence and self-esteem. As Yates and Boddison state in *The School Handbook for Dual and Multiple Exceptionality*,[20]

Focusing on the gifts, talents and interests of children with DME (whilst accommodating their difficulties) is more likely to result in improved resilience and the experience of success. If they are given opportunities to develop their strengths, these children can develop a positive image of who they are and a vision of what they might become.

Collaboration and communication

Collaboration and communication are essential in supporting children with DME/2e. In fact the DME Trust report[21] called for this as one of the things that would help children with DME the most. Parents, teachers and other professionals should work together to ensure that the child's needs are being met. This involves regular communication between parents and teachers, and collaboration between different professionals, such as occupational therapists, speech therapists and psychologists.

Opportunities to build relationships with peers

One of the five areas of support for children with DME/2e that Beverly Trail addresses in her book *Twice-Exceptional Gifted Children: Understanding, Teaching and Counseling Gifted Students* (2022)[22] is fostering relationships. As Howell puts it in her article "Best Practice in Provision for Dual or Multiple Exceptional (DME) Learners" (2020),[23] "Strong, positive relationships with peers, parents and other adults are important for every child and a significant factor for academic success. They are vital for DME learners with asynchronous development, which is often misunderstood".

Of particular importance is building positive relationships with peers to reduce feelings of isolation. This can be achieved through social skills groups, extracurricular activities and other social opportunities. However, it's important to approach these opportunities in a way that is sensitive to the child's needs and challenges. For example, a child who has anxiety challenges may benefit from smaller group settings or one-on-one social interactions. As well as promoting positive social interactions, parents and educators need to be aware of and guard against bullying.

Awareness of underachievement

Finally, parents and educators should be aware of the potential for underachievement in children with DME/2e. Due to their challenges and the barriers they face in finding appropriate support, children with DME/2e are at significant risk of underachieving or disengaging from their education. As Falck (2020) explains:

> When gifted individuals are in an environment where very little effort is needed from them to stay abreast of the level of achievement that is expected of them and being demonstrated by their peers, they do not acquire the habit of disciplined, persistent effort that is necessary to accomplish anything of real importance (Hollingworth 1942;

Towers 1987; Grobman 2006). Developing lazy habits means that if they later find themselves facing challenges that they are unable to meet with little effort, they either avoid the challenge, or fail at it. The former establishes a pattern of underachievement, while the latter can be experienced as devastating because the praise they have received for their prior effortless achievements builds an identity as an achiever that they can become dependent on for their self-esteem and which is then threatened.

It is therefore important for parents and educators to monitor the progress of children with DME/2e and provide support as needed to ensure they are meeting their academic and social potential.

The Portrayal of DME/2e in the Media

When the topic of HLP or giftedness is portrayed in the media, it is often represented as a positive characteristic only. Individuals with HLP are regularly depicted as high achievers who are destined for success. However, as previously discussed, the reality is that being gifted can come with its own set of challenges, and this is particularly so for those with DME/2e. When people with DME/2e are portrayed in the media, the unique challenges they face and their experiences are often overlooked; they are frequently painted in a negative light. For example, people with DME/2e are portrayed with traits such as laziness, uncooperativeness or even disruptiveness. This can lead to further stigmatisation and can be harmful to the self-esteem of children with DME/2e. It can also lead to a lack of understanding and support for their needs.

There have been some recent efforts to raise awareness about DME/2e in the media. For example, in the television show *Atypical*, the main character is an autistic teenager who is also gifted in mathematics. While the show has received criticism for some aspects of its portrayal of autism, it has been praised for its depiction of the challenges faced by individuals with DME/2e. Another example of DME/2e representation in the media is the documentary *2e: Twice Exceptional*. This film explores the lives of children with DME/2e and their families, highlighting their struggles and successes. It also features interviews with experts in the field, providing valuable insight into the experiences of children with DME/2e.

The 2017 film *Gifted* is a heartwarming family story that depicts a young girl with high learning potential and the tensions her family undergoes in trying to raise her. In the backstory, we find that her mother had also been gifted but had mental health struggles (placing her in the DME/2e category). The girl's uncle fights to make sure history does not repeat itself. The 2016 film *The Accountant* features Ben Affleck as an autistic man with "more affinity for numbers than people" according to the blurb about the film on the Warner Brothers website. Behind the cover of a small accountancy firm, he works as a freelance accountant for some of the world's most dangerous criminal organisations. The 2014 film *The Imitation Game* is based on the life of legendary cryptanalyst Alan Turing who was widely believed to be autistic and so would have had a DME/2e profile.

One of the most famous, and indeed the first, instances of a DME/2e character in the media was in the 1988 film *Rain Man*, in which Dustin Hoffman plays an autistic savant. However, the depiction led to public misunderstandings about autism since many thought that all autistic people had amazing abilities like those portrayed in the movie, whereas in reality many autistic people do not. Despite not being malicious in its portrayal, the film is thought to be a poor representation and a stereotype of autistic people.

In *The Chosen*, an American Christian drama series about the life of Jesus, the tax-collecting disciple Matthew is portrayed as someone who is DME/2e, gifted and autistic. In 2012/2013 the American drama series *Touch* starred Kiefer Sutherland as a single dad raising his autistic son who is fascinated by numbers and patterns relating to numbers, spending much of his days writing them down in notebooks or his touch-screen tablet. *A Beautiful Mind* is an American biographical film about the life of John Nash, a Nobel Laureate in Economics who was a brilliant mathematician and was diagnosed with schizophrenia.

Overall, while there have been some efforts to raise awareness about people with DME/2e in the media, there is still a long way to go. Portraying children with DME/2e in a more accurate and positive light, highlighting their strengths and abilities while also acknowledging their challenges, would reduce stereotyping and stigma and increase understanding and support them and their families.

Well Known People with DME/2e

In real life, children with DME/2e do have some great role models though. A handful of people with neurodiversity and disabilities that would likely have a DME/2e profile are outlined below. However, readers will now in all probability be able to identify many more well known people with DME/2e in their own cultures and communities.

- **Greta Thunberg**, a Swedish environmental activist known for challenging world leaders to take immediate action for climate change mitigation from the age of 15, is autistic and has obsessive compulsive disorder
- **Daniel Radcliffe**, the English actor who rose to fame at the age of 12 playing Harry Potter in the films of the same name, has dyspraxia
- **Octavia Spencer** is an Academy Award-winning actress and author who has dyslexia
- **Steven Spielberg**, the most commercially successful filmmaker in history, also has dyslexia
- **Stephen Hawking**, theoretical physicist, cosmologist and mathematician, had motor neuron disease. In fact, in 2018, Stephen Hawking launched the National Association of Special Educational Needs' work on DME/2e at their annual conference, nasen Live!
- **John Nash**, the American Nobel Laureate for Economics who made fundamental contributions to game theory, real algebraic geometry, differential geometry and partial differential equations, had a diagnosis of schizophrenia

- **Richard Branson**, English billionaire and philanthropist who founded the Virgin Group, has dyslexia
- **David Beckham** OBE, the English former professional footballer, has obsessive compulsive disorder
- It is widely believed that **Albert Einstein**, German-born theoretical physicist who developed the theory of relativity, was autistic
- It is widely accepted that **Alan Turing**, English mathematician and pioneer of theoretical computer science and artificial intelligence who broke the Enigma code during the second world war, was autistic
- **Michael Phelps**, American swimmer and the most successful and decorated Olympian of all time, has ADHD
- **Maggie Aderin-Pocock** MBE, British space scientist and science educator, has dyslexia
- **Anne Hegarty**, one of the "chasers" on the British ITV game show *The Chase*, known as The Governess on the show, is autistic
- **Simone Biles**, the most decorated gymnast in the history of the Gymnastics World Championships, has ADHD. She is considered by many sources to be the greatest gymnast of all time
- **Daryl Hannah**, American actress and environmental activist, is autistic
- **Tom Cruise**, one of the highest paid American actors and film producer, is dyslexic

Conclusion

This chapter built on the understanding about high learning potential/giftedness gained in Chapter 2. Whilst it is difficult to generalise about children with DME/2e because their profiles vary so much depending on their special educational need or disability, this chapter gave readers some understanding about these children with a view to being able to identify them in their practice. Key to this is understanding the strengths and deficits of the individual child as well as their asynchronous development.

Once a child with DME/2e is identified as such, the adults around them need to have an awareness of the barriers they face, what scenarios they find themselves in and the support they may need to thrive. It can also be helpful to see how DME/2e is portrayed in the media and what role models children with DME/2e have.

In Chapter 4 we outline the general SEND diagnoses that children with DME/2e have and pinpoint which of these occupational therapists are best suited to address.

Notes

* Special Educational Need or Disability (SEND) is the term used in England to describe children or young people who have a learning difficulty or disability which calls for special educational provision to be made for him or her.
† nasen is the National Association for Special Educational Needs in the UK.

References

1. Kircher-Morris, E. (2020, August 19) Episode 65: A Talk with a 2e Pioneer. *The Neurodiversity Podcast*. https://neurodiversitypodcast.com/home/2020/8/19/episode-65-a-talk-with-a-2e-pioneer.
2. Tetreault, N. A. (2021) *Insight into a Bright Mind: A Neuroscientist's Personal Stories of Unique Thinking*. Gifted Unlimited.
3. Montgomery, D. (2015) *Teaching Gifted Children with SEN: Supporting Dual and Multiple Exceptionality*. Routledge.
4. Department for Children, Schools and Families. (2008). The National Strategies. *Gifted and talented education: Helping to find and support children with dual or multiple exceptionalities*. DCFS Publications. Available at: https://webarchive.nationalarchives.gov.uk/20130323073730/https:/www.education.gov.uk/publications/eOrderingDownload/00052-2008BKT-EN.pdf.
5. Kircher-Morris, E. (2022) *Raising Twice-Exceptional Children: A Handbook for Parents of Neurodivergent Gifted Kids*. Prufrock Press.
6. Ronksley-Pavia, Michelle. (2014). *Understanding Twice-exceptionality: Children with Disability and Giftedness*. 10.13140/2.1.4602.1446.
7. Gagné, Françoys. (2012). Building talent on the foundations of giftedness: Overview of the DMGT 2.0. *ANAE - Approche Neuropsychologique des Apprentissages chez l'Enfant*. 24. 409-417.
8. Ryan, A., & Waterman. C. (2018). *Dual & Multiple Exceptionality (DME): The current state of play*. nasen https://asset.nasen.org.uk/DME-Stateof-play-.pdf.
9. McDonald, B., Lester, K. & Michelson, D. (2023) 'She didn't know how to go back': School attendance problems in the context of the COVID-19 pandemic—A multiple stakeholder qualitative study with parents and professionals. *British Journal of Educational Psychology*, 93(1) https://doi.org/10.1111/bjep.12562.
10. Higgins, L. D., & Nielsen, M. E. (2000). Teaching the twice-exceptional child: An educator's personal journey. In Kay K. (Ed.), *Uniquely gifted: Identifying and meeting the needs of the twice-exceptional student* (pp. 113-131). Gilsum, NH: Avocus.
11. Potential Plus UK (2019) F01 Dual or Multiple Exceptionality (DME). [Fact Sheet]
12. Center on the Developing Child (n.d.) Executive Function & Self-Regulation. https://developingchild.harvard.edu/science/key-concepts/executive-function/.
13. Beck, C. (2021, July 8) *Emotional Regulation and Executive Function*. The OT Toolbox. https://www.theottoolbox.com/emotional-regulation-and-executive-function/.
14. Butnik, S. (2020) *Understanding, Diagnosing and Coping with Slow Processing Speed*. Davidson Institute. https://www.davidsongifted.org/gifted-blog/understanding-diagnosing-and-coping-with-slow-processing-speed/.
15. Bonsall, A. & Desmond, B. (2022) *The Current State of Provision for Learners with DME*. The DME Trust. https://potentialplusuk.org/wp-content/uploads/2022/01/220110-DME-The-Current-State-of-Provision-Report.pdf.
16. Falck, S. (2020) *Extreme Intelligence: Development, Predicaments, Implications*. Routledge.
17. Potential Plus UK (2019) F01 Dual or Multiple Exceptionality (DME). [Fact Sheet]
18. Wormald, C., Rogers, K. & Vialle, W. (2015). A Case Study of Giftedness and Specific Learning Disabilities: Bridging the Two Exceptionalities. Roeper Review. 37. 124-138.
19. Hirt, K. (2018) *Boost: 12 Effective Ways to Lift Up Our Twice-Exceptional Children*. GHF Press.
20. Yates, D. & Boddison, A. (2020) *The School Handbook for Dual and Multiple Exceptionality: High Learning Potential with Special Educational Needs or Disabilities*. Routledge.
21. Bonsall, A. & Desmond, B. (2022) The Current State of Provision for Learners with DME. The DME Trust. https://potentialplusuk.org/wp-content/uploads/2022/01/220110-DME-The-Current-State-of-Provision-Report.pdf.
22. Trail, B. A. (2022) *Twice-Exceptional Gifted Children: Understanding, Teaching, and Counseling Gifted Students* (2nd Edition). Routledge.
23. Howell, R. (2020, January 13) Best Practice in Provision for Dual or Multiple Exceptional (DME) Learners. *Whole School SEND*. https://www.wholeschoolsend.org.uk/blog/ppuk-best-practice-provision-dual-or-multiple-exceptional-dme-learners

Chapter four
DME/Twice Exceptionality and Occupational Therapy

Introduction

The most common[1] SEND that children with high learning potential have include but are not limited to:

- Autism, usually diagnosed as autism spectrum disorder/condition (ASD/ASC)
- Attention deficit hyperactivity disorder (ADHD)
- Developmental coordination disorder (DCD) including dyspraxia
- Dyslexia, dysgraphia, dyscalculia
- Sensory processing difficulties
- Visual and hearing impairments
- Other physical disabilities
- Speech and language delays or impairments
- Social, emotional, mental health issues and behavioural difficulties

Paediatric occupational therapists can help children with high learning potential and DME/2e with challenges related to all of these conditions and profiles and, for ease of reference for the purposes of this chapter, we can categorise the children into three groups.

Group 1 – Developmental and neurological differences

The first group is the children occupational therapists most commonly see in general or "mainstream" paediatric practice and are those who have a confirmed diagnosis or are suspected of having autism spectrum disorder, attention deficit hyperactivity disorder, developmental coordination disorder including dyspraxia, dysgraphia (or to avoid confusion – handwriting difficulties) and sensory processing difficulties or differences. We will discuss all these profiles and how they relate to high learning potential later in this chapter, apart from sensory processing differences which we will discuss in Chapter 5.

Group 2 – Sensory impairments and complex physical needs

The second group of children are the ones for whom their challenges relate to the functioning of their physical bodies, resulting in significant difficulties with everyday life tasks. This is when children have sensory impairments and complex physical needs such as visual and/or hearing impairments, cerebral palsy, muscular dystrophy or epilepsy and speech and

DOI: 10.4324/9781003334033-4

language delays or impairments. Although, occupational therapists mostly work in collaboration with speech and language therapists in the case of the latter. In the UK this group of children will undoubtedly already be known to statutory services and occupational therapists in dedicated physical disability teams.

It is a given that the main occupational therapy for these children will revolve around meeting their functional needs of personal care such as eating, getting dressed, personal hygiene, education, accessing education and leisure and play with access to these. Therapy is mostly focused on the provision of bespoke home and school adaptations, both minor and major in nature, to ensure they are accessible for the disabled child; the provision of assistive technology in the form of equipment, devices and software such as eating aids, hoists and slings for safe moving and handling, specialist wheelchairs, adapted computer keyboards and dictation software to name but a few; and adapted or alternative ways to play games and allow for social interaction such as the use of single switch entry devices.

It is vital to help children with high learning potential and physical disabilities become as independent as possible in their daily lives, but when the focus is mainly on their SEND, there is the risk that their high learning ability or potential is overlooked or not catered for effectively.

Whilst it is not the job of occupational therapists to provide a child with an education, therapists are often in ideal positions to recognise when a child with physical disabilities also has high learning potential, which means therapists can liaise with the necessary professionals and advocate for the child's high learning potential to be accommodated alongside their physical disabilities or SEND.

Furthermore, as occupational therapists learn more about high learning potential and DME/2e, and the unique issues that this group of children face, therapists can adapt their own methods of providing therapy to make them more strengths-based and effective. For instance, if a child with DME/2e with restricted motor skills has a keen eye for design, the occupational therapist can ensure that the child is actively involved in the process of planning and designing the decor of their newly adapted room with the use of assistive technology.

Group 3 – Social, emotional and mental health needs

The third group of children are the ones who have social, emotional, mental health issues and behavioural difficulties. Occupational therapists who work in dedicated children's mental health services, such as Child and Adolescent Mental Health Services (CAMHS), are well-placed to help children with high learning potential and mental health difficulties who qualify for services. However, this set of challenges is not exclusive to children who qualify for help from mental health services. In fact, social, emotional and/or mental health needs are often present across the board in the children with high learning potential and DME/2e that occupational therapists work with. However, because these needs arise as a result of other factors such as sensory or motor skills deficits, children who experience these challenges do not qualify for CAMHS input, and working with them through "mainstream" paediatric occupational therapy is sometimes the only way they can receive help to address some of their social, emotional and mental health needs.

For example, children with high learning potential who have developmental coordination disorder (DCD) may have low self-esteem because they are unable to do up their shoelaces during physical education lessons in school. This difficulty may cause others, such as teachers or their peers, to misunderstand them and label them as "difficult", "lazy" or "uninterested" in a lesson. When therapists help these children find strategies to tie their shoelaces independently and successfully, it will automatically improve their self-esteem, sense of achievement and thereby their perceived attitude.

Similarly, children with high learning potential and sensory processing differences, such as tactile defensiveness, who have adverse and aggressive reactions when others accidentally touch them when queuing up for class, will develop better self-awareness and more appropriate coping strategies with the help of occupational therapy. This in turn will improve their social skills and acceptance amongst their peers.

There are certain times when occupational therapists may help address children with high learning potential's social, emotional, mental health and behavioural difficulties without these difficulties having an apparent root cause in a motor and/or sensory skills deficit. Rather, the causes for their social, emotional, mental health and behavioural difficulties seem to be rooted in some of the common characteristics of children with HLP, as reported by their parents (see Chapter 2), including asynchronous development and social isolation. For example, children with HLP and their families may seek occupational therapy to help them cope better with the intense emotions and adverse emotional reactions they experience on a continual basis in response to their own circumstances and world events that other children may take no or little notice of. We call these root causes the "non-occupational therapy factors" (or "non-OT factors"), as they relate more directly to high learning potential than areas of difficulties traditionally addressed through occupational therapy, such as sensory or motor skills deficits and challenges, and associated difficulties with emotional self-regulation (the "OT-factors"). It is important to note that occupational therapists can work with children with HLP whose social, emotional, mental health and behavioural difficulties are rooted in the non-OT factors only, but more often than not occupational therapists work with children whose difficulties stem from both non-OT and OT-factors.

In the next paragraph we discuss the non-OT factors further, as it is important for therapists to actively consider these in their work with children with HLP and DME/2e.

The Non-OT Factors

By way of a reminder, the term non-OT factors refers to some of the common characteristics that children with HLP across the world share, including asynchronous development and social isolation. These can cause children with HLP and DME/2e to have social, emotional, mental health and behavioural difficulties and/or these can impact on therapy. We briefly discuss the characteristics of perfectionism, fear of failure, fixed mindset, acute social awareness, empathy and sense of right and wrong, intellectual boredom, tendency to question authority, asynchronous development and social isolation later in this section. Therapists should be mindful that because the impact of the common characteristics could be positive as well as negative, such as the child having the ability to learn rapidly during the therapy process or a child having an acute social awareness motivating them to engage in community projects, we include **all** the common characteristics under the umbrella term of non-OT factors.

Children with high learning potential and DME/2e often have strong tendencies to lean towards **perfectionism,**[2] a **fear of failure** and, hand in hand with that, a **fixed mindset**. A child may have a very specific idea of what their drawing should look like but when their artistic skills and fine motor pencil control do not live up to the task of producing the picture they had in their head, they are at risk of internalising this failure and developing a fixed mindset of "I am bad at art". This could also lead to a fear of failure when faced with similar activities in the future, and often an outright refusal to engage with any task that remotely resembles "art".

Similarly, children with high learning potential often have an **acute social awareness, empathy** and **sense of right and wrong** when it comes to local or even world events that may not concern other children their age. They are often deeply offended when a teacher tells them off for doing something wrong and then weeks later does not tell off another child for doing something which they perceive as the same as their own. Also, these children are often so aware, disturbed and sometimes depressed by world events that they cannot see the point of carrying on with their everyday or "normal" activities such as school, sport or clubs, when they feel they should be doing something to help and change the situation, even though they may be thousands of miles away from it. One example of this was when working with a six-year-old child with DME/2e at the time we started becoming aware of Covid-19 early in 2020. The child was so worried about the effect of the pandemic on a global scale that it was impossible to continue with the session until the therapist had acknowledged and addressed the child's fears.

Another non-OT issue that children with DME/2e often have is that they are not challenged adequately on a cognitive level and find themselves **intellectually bored** at school. This often leads to challenging and unacceptable behaviour. For example, the mother of a young child explained that he once swiped all the papers and writing equipment off his table and onto the floor whilst the teacher was explaining what the class had to do. This child had severe auditory sensitivities, and at first the therapist thought it was because the class was perhaps too noisy on that occasion. However, once the therapist worked with the child and they explored coping strategies together, he revealed that he swiped the materials off the table as he was highly frustrated with how easy the work was that they had to do and that he felt the teacher was wasting his time. He was five and a half at the time...

It can be hard for teachers, parents and professionals to spot intellectual boredom as a core reason for a child's unacceptable behaviours. This is especially tough considering that children with high learning potential and DME/2e sometimes struggle with more mundane academic tasks such as simple adding and subtracting in class. Yet, at home in their spare time, they like doing much more complex mathematics in their heads! At school they may sometimes show no interest in reading the age-appropriate books which form part of the curriculum, leading educators to believe that they are behind with their reading; whilst at home they have read a whole series of much more advanced material.

It is understandable and quite common to hear educators say it is impossible for a child to be "bright" or have a particular strength in a subject area when they have not seen any evidence of it in class. In fact, they may have only observed the opposite. The danger of continued misidentification of a child's true academic potential and ability, and/or lack of accommodating it when identified by the significant adults in their life, is that the child develops a mistrust of these people in particular and perhaps authority figures in general. This can lead to the child giving up trying to prove himself and his abilities or potential to achieve, disengaging from schoolwork and, in extreme cases, becoming a school refuser.

One parent's experience of how her child's intellectual boredom was affecting his education:

"The school believed my son to be autistic and explained away his early reading, love of numbers and shapes this way. They later refuted that he could have HLP as he was 'behind' in class and to this day they can only record him being at the level they see. This is a kid who wrote in Russian at two years of age.

I only found out about 'gifted' kids when I googled his so-called 'class behaviours' where some teachers said he was silent and did not engage, and other teachers said he never stopped asking questions.

The school paid for an educational psychologist report as they believed he was autistic. I believed gifted or 2e. The report came back plain old gifted/HLP.

Lots and lots of strategies were recommended but none have been implemented. Yet I am told, 'He daydreams, he moves in and out of his seat, he is not naughty, but he just seems to switch off". I have pushed back with intellectual boredom as a reason, especially with the backup of the massive educational psychology report, but the school feels the report must be wrong. They have referred him to the local autism service.

My child is literally saying he is bored, but in school he looks at the work, ignores it and says, 'It is too hard'. He cannot articulate to them that it is **too hard for him to focus on as it is so basic and he is so bored**.

I now pay for private tutoring sessions. His tutor reports he does not fidget, he is polite, he is engaged and always shocked when the lesson is up. He is not at all bored, and ahead of his chronological age in his level of skill. I did not tell the tutor he was gifted on starting. She told me by the end of the first lesson.

Boredom is a real killer. It's not always sensory processing differences. It is not always autism. Sometimes it is one, the other, or neither".

Since working with children with high learning potential and DME/2e, especially at the start of the intervention process, we have learnt to always be very conscious of the fact that these children may be harbouring a hidden distrust of authority figures, ourselves included. This, together with their high cognitive ability and related tendency to **question authority** in general, is often a recipe for confrontation at some point in the therapy process. The children will either try to hide their true feelings, with resistance to participation in therapy sessions and engagement with therapy homework between sessions increasing over time, which we call the "slow burner". Or they may be very vocal and openly resistant to input from the start, which we refer to as the "instant explosion". Dealing with this as a therapist, and ultimately breaking through the resistive barrier with distrust at its foundation, is not an easy task in either of these cases. But it is essential and highly rewarding to gain a child's trust so that therapy can be effective and bring about lasting change in the child's life.

Occupational therapists also need to be aware of the effect of **asynchronous development** on the social and emotional development of a child. We know that children with high learning potential often have the spiky profile of being very advanced in certain areas but delayed with others. This can relate to certain subjects e.g. a child can be significantly ahead of their peers in maths, but behind with English. Equally, a child can be ahead of their peers academically in general, but be emotionally immature to the point where their behaviours are rejected by their peers. In this case the child who is already singled out for being "too smart for their own good", is avoided as others may find it just too hard to play games with them or socialise with them.

Social isolation and feeling alone is probably one of biggest non-OT factors (and problems) for a child with high learning potential and DME/2e. During all the meetings and conferences we have attended over the years with parents of and professionals working with children with high learning potential and DME/2e, from not just the UK but all over Europe as well, the universal concern that is always discussed at length is social isolation and the impact it has on the mental health of the children. This is why it is important to support children to develop a sense of belonging, in whatever way is possible for them.

The importance of a sense of belonging

In our opinion and experience, having a sense of belonging whilst feeling comfortable in one's own skin, perhaps more than "fitting in", is one of the most important needs of a child with high learning potential and DME/2e. When a child feels they belong, they can confidently be themselves without needing to try and hide their strengths or weaknesses. They are accepted for who they are, and they will ultimately be a happier child who is more likely to achieve their full potential.

In contrast, a child who is trying to fit in may adopt behaviours prevalent of the crowd they are trying to fit into, hide how smart they are, even deliberately do poorly in tests, and hide their real emotions. This child may initially be happy to be part of the crowd, but with time they are likely to feel more unfulfilled and experience growing unhappiness. It will be harder for this child to reach their full potential.

Helping a socially isolated child to achieve a feeling or sense of belonging is complicated but possible. It means using all the tools available from the occupational therapy set of skills or toolbox, and often it involves thinking outside the box and following a "therapeutic gut instinct". As therapists, we can address many aspects that will help a child feel like they belong, but at the same time it is essential to know that we cannot achieve this on our own, nor does it fall only in our remit or scope. This is why collaborative working and ongoing clear communication with a child's parents, teachers and other relevant professionals is essential.

Why the non-OT factors are important

Regardless of whether children with high learning potential and DME/2e are in mainly one or from across the three groups mentioned above, it is important to be aware of the non-OT factors that could be affecting them, so therapists can adapt the method in which they provide therapy for these children to ensure it remains strengths-based. To support and empower therapists in this, we offer the "10 Golden Nuggets" of the DME-C therapy approach (see Chapter 6). While not all the 10 Golden Nuggets are applicable for children across groups one to three, many of the nuggets are indeed relevant.

For now it will suffice to highlight the importance of following the occupational therapy process with each child with DME/2e, which starts with a thorough assessment of both the child's strengths and challenges as a means to get an holistic picture of the child. This will help set realistic and achievable therapy goals with children and their families, direct the therapy itself by making it easier for occupational therapists to determine which therapy approaches to use, and help to identify the need for other professional input to signpost or refer the child as appropriate.

A Closer Look at Occupational Therapy for Children in Group 1 – Developmental and Neurological Differences

Whilst we will mainly focus on children with high learning potential or DME/2e who have sensory processing differences in this book, we do think it is important to also look at some of the accompanying conditions and profiles or special educational needs or disabilities (SEND) that these children could have, and that we often see in mainstream paediatric occupational therapy.

It would be possible to write a book on each one of the SENDs and how best to work in therapy with children in general who face related challenges. In fact, as is well-known, there are already hundreds of books on these topics – not just within occupational therapy but within other healthcare professions as well. We will therefore only provide a snapshot of each SEND, starting with its definition and how it relates to high learning potential and DME/2e, including similarities and differences. We will follow this with a brief discussion on the best approaches, in our opinion, to help children with high learning potential who have these conditions or profiles. In Chapter 5 we will look in more detail at sensory processing differences in children with high learning potential and DME/2e.

Developmental Coordination Disorder (DCD), Including Dyspraxia

Definition

DCD[3] is a motor skills disorder that affects between 5 to 6% of school-aged children and is a lifelong condition. It affects a person's fine and/or gross motor coordination, with the person having severe difficulties coordinating their movements sufficiently to consistently perform everyday motor skills successfully, and/or in the learning of new and age-related everyday motor skills. These difficulties cannot be explained by physical, sensory or intellectual impairments and occur across a range of intellectual abilities. DCD affects a range of activities across all the spheres of a person's life: personal care and self-management, work or school and leisure. A few examples are difficulties with dressing, eating with cutlery, handwriting, typing, working with tools, riding a bicycle and playing sports. There may be a range of co-occurring difficulties which can negatively impact on a person's life, such as social and emotional difficulties as well as problems with time management and organisation.

DCD is formally recognised by international organisations including the World Health Organisation. The full criteria for the diagnosis of DCD is listed in the *Diagnostic and Statistical Manual of Mental Disorders, Fifth Edition* (DSM-V) and the *International Statistical Classification of Diseases and Related Health Problems* (ICD-11).

It is important to note that in some countries such as the USA, people use the term "dyspraxia" as a substitute for DCD, or the two terms are used interchangeably. Whilst this has also been the case in the UK for some years, there is a consistent move among professionals towards using the term DCD instead, in part because it is a recognised standalone condition whereas dyspraxia is not.

When considering the term dyspraxia,[4] which can be explained as a difficulty to plan, organise and carry out a sequence of unfamiliar actions and to do what one needs to do or wants to do, it is easy to see how it forms part of a diagnosis of DCD. However, dyspraxia is also classified under the umbrella term of sensory processing disorder, subtype sensory based motor disorder,[5] especially in the USA. Occupational therapists need to be mindful of these differences in terminology when working with children with DME/2e with DCD, as well as their families and teachers, to ensure any confusion is cleared up and allow everyone to focus on helping the child.

High learning potential and DCD

Children with DCD tend to have high verbal IQs.[6] With regards to the performance of motor tasks, there is no difference in the clinical presentation between children with DCD who have high learning potential (DME) and typical children with DCD.[7] However, the children with DME/2e appear to have better executive functioning and visio-spatial functioning, but worse auditory attention and memory then typical children with DCD. This suggests that the children with DME/2e may have better planning abilities to work through motor tasks as they use more visual representations and internal language than typical children with DCD, but they cannot rely so much on remembering the steps of a task when given only verbally.

With regards to tasks which primarily require gross motor skills, children with DME/2e and DCD may decide not to engage in any form of sport, or they may choose to participate in a sport where they can control the environment. For instance, they may choose (and be very good at!) track athletics or playing golf instead of off-road running, skiing, football or tennis where the environment is fast or constantly changing.

With regards to tasks that involve fine motor skills, especially in a school context, these children most commonly struggle with handwriting speed and legibility but also with personal care tasks such as tying shoelaces or doing up the buttons on their shirts.

It is also interesting to consider that children with DME/2e who have DCD may struggle with their handwriting due to joint hypermobility syndrome or Ehlers-Danlos Syndrome, which affects each child to varying degrees, and which contributes to the physical task of handwriting being effortful and painful. It has been suggested[8] that there is a higher occurrence of Ehlers-Danlos Syndrome in people who have high learning potential than those considered to be without it.

Note about some non-OT factors that may influence handwriting:

Children with high learning potential sometimes may not have a physical or cognitive difficulty with handwriting. Instead, it could be that their writing hand just cannot keep up with their own fast, free flowing and innovative ideas. They may be reluctant to write or have a tendency to write slowly despite much encouragement from therapists, parents or teachers. This is because of their perfectionistic traits and fear of making a mistake. Mariza, one of the authors, saw this particularly with one child during an occupational therapy assessment. She asked him to write for ten minutes on a topic of his choice and presented him with a range of ideas similar to those given by the DASH (Detailed Assessment of Speed of Handwriting UK standardised test). However, the child "froze", and showed signs of distress by his breathing becoming rapid and his face becoming red. He needed guidance and support to calm down and was able to complete the task with encouragement. After the assessment, the child informed Mariza that part of the reason for him freezing was that he was afraid to "make the wrong choice" about which topic to choose.

Best therapy approach to help children with HLP and difficulties related to DCD

We know that occupational therapists have different and sometimes contradicting opinions on the best approaches to help children with DCD and other motor skills related difficulties. Some therapists prefer bottom-up approaches such as using Ayres Sensory Integration® (ASI), and others prefer top-down approaches such as the Cognitive Orientation to Daily Occupational Performance (CO-OP/CO-OP Approach)™. Our preference is to use top-down approaches such as the CO-OP, or elements thereof as part of an eclectic and bespoke approach, when the main difficulty a child with DME/2e wants to work on relates to motor skills tasks. This is because any input involving cognitive strategies are likely to go much further with children with DME/2e, as they love thinking things through, and this is especially the case when the goal is to solve problems. Whichever approach therapists choose, our encouragement would be to ensure it is compatible with the information and guidance shared in this book.

The CO-OP[9] was developed by Helene J. Polatajko and Angela Mandich and is a client-centred, performance-based, problem solving approach that enables skill acquisition. It is focussed on enabling success through the process of collaborative goal setting, dynamic performance analysis, cognitive strategy use, guided discovery and enabling principles which are considered essential to the CO-OP. Working with children to find strategies they feel comfortable with not only improves their current task performance but it also helps them to develop an overall problem-solving strategy for new tasks in the future.

Therapists can find out more information about how to become certified CO-OP practitioners, by visiting the official website on https://icancoop.org.

Autism or Autistic Spectrum Disorder (ASD)*

Definition

Autism or Autism Spectrum Disorder[10,11,12] affects approximately 1 in 100 children worldwide, and 700,000 people in the UK, and is a lifelong neurodevelopmental condition. Autistic people have different communication styles and preferences, and persistent difficulties with neurotypical social communication and social interaction, often display stereotypical (rigid and repetitive) behaviour, experience sensory under or over responsiveness to the environment, have highly focussed and/or restricted interests or hobbies, are resistant to change and can experience intense anxiety.

The level of intellectual functioning among autistic people can range from profound impairment, or learning disability as it is known in the UK, to having high learning potential or being 'gifted'. Formerly autistic children and adults with relatively unimpaired language or intelligence were referred to as having Asperger's Disorder[13] or Syndrome. This term is no longer a subcategory of autism and this group is included under the umbrella term.

Autism affects people in different ways. Some autistic people can live independently whilst others need lifetime care and support. Autism can have a marked impact on all the spheres of a person's life: personal care and self-management, work or school, and leisure. By way of further explanation, the particular common difficulties autistic people may experience are described in the next few paragraphs.

With regards to communication, autistic people have difficulties with interpreting verbal and non-verbal language like gestures or tone of voice. They can be non-verbal or have limited speech, or they can have good language skills but struggle to understand sarcasm or tone of voice. Autistic people typically take words literally and need extra time to process information or answer questions, or they may repeat what others say to them (echolalia).

When it comes to social interaction, autistic people have difficulty 'reading' others such as understanding their feelings and intentions, as well as expressing their own emotions. This can make them appear insensitive when in fact they care a lot about others. They will seek out time alone when they feel overloaded by social situations, not seek comfort from others, appear to behave "strangely" or inappropriately in social situations at times, and may find it hard to form or sustain friendships.

Autistic people often display stereotypical (rigid and repetitive) behaviour. They have a strong preference for routines so that they can know what is going to happen e.g. always wanting to eat the same food for breakfast. They often repeat movements such as hand flapping, rocking or closing a door which is also referred to as 'stimming behaviour', as it helps them to feel calm when stressed or anxious or because they find the actual behaviour enjoyable.

Another characteristic is that autistic people often experience sensory over responsiveness or sensory overload depending on the environment. This mostly refers to sounds, touch, tastes, smells, light, colours, temperature or pain. They will therefore try to avoid these sensory experiences by staying away from public places such as schools, shopping centres or workplaces.

Autistic people often have intense and highly focussed and or restricted interests or hobbies, which can change over time or be lifelong. They can become experts in their specialist interest and often like to share their knowledge with others. Like all people, autistic people gain pleasure from pursuing their interests and see them as fundamental to their wellbeing and happiness. Autistic people can therefore do very well academically and in the workplace, but being engrossed by particular topics can both support and be at the expense of other areas of their lives.

Many autistic children (and adults) can struggle with anxiety and become distressed in social situations or when dealing with change such as being expected to follow a different routine, having an unexpected teacher for the day or going on holiday to somewhere unfamiliar. They often have difficulty regulating their emotions and can experience mental health issues as a result.

When 'things become too much' for autistic children, such as when they experience sensory overload at school, in shopping centres and even in the workplace, they can go into a meltdown which could be verbal such as shouting or crying, physical such as lashing out or biting, or both. In children this can often be mistaken for a temper tantrum. They can also go into shutdown which looks like they are 'switching off' but their internal experience and feelings are no less intense.

Autism is formally recognised by international organisations including the World Health Organisation. The full criteria for the diagnosis of Autism is listed in the *Diagnostic and Statistical Manual of Mental Disorders, Fifth Edition* (DSM-V) and the *International Statistical Classification of Diseases and Related Health Problems* (ICD-11).

High learning potential and autism

Becoming familiar with what autism is and how it presents in children will help therapists to recognise associated difficulties and support autistic children better. This can be done by visiting websites such as The National Autistic Society https://www.autism.org.uk/, which is the leading UK based charity supporting autistic people and their families, and doing training courses on the topic specifically designed for occupational therapists. There are many similarities between autism and high learning potential, which can lead to children with the latter being misdiagnosed with autism. However, it is possible for children to be autistic and have high learning potential, in which case they have the profile of DME/2e. Of course, all these groups of children often have additional challenges such as sensory processing differences, just to add to the mix.

Similarities

Two examples of traits that are similar between autistic children and those with high learning potential are that both groups of children may appear socially awkward and have excellent memories for facts. However, the reason an autistic child appears socially awkward is because they struggle with neurotypical social interaction and reading social cues. Alternatively, a child with high learning potential has advanced cognitive thinking patterns as opposed to their peers, making it difficult to find a connection point or common ground with children their age. Furthermore, both sets of children may have an excellent memory for facts. A child with high learning potential will often be able to apply this to a variety of topics, whereas an autistic child mostly applies this ability to the areas of their specific interests or hobbies.

For the purposes of clarification, a child can be solely on the autism spectrum, have high learning potential on its own, or have a profile combining the two together, in which case they have the profile of DME/2e. However, a child with high learning potential can also be misdiagnosed as autistic if the professionals in the assessment and diagnostic team have not considered the child's cognitive abilities through suitable specialist assessments, either done by themselves or by another appropriate professional or organisation.

The more information there is about a child's strengths and challenges, the more therapists will be able to help the child. Occupational therapists who are part of an autism assessment and diagnostic team for children are encouraged to consider or highlight the necessity of formally exploring a child's cognitive and intellectual ability further where it is suspected that high learning potential may be part of the child's profile. Occupational therapists are often the only professionals who are in a position to view a child holistically, so it is important to speak up even if it turns out to be an unfounded suspicion with regards to their cognitive ability.

Occupational therapists working in mainstream paediatric occupational therapy may see children who already have a diagnosis of autism, or the children's parents or teachers may look towards occupational therapists for guidance on whether the child could be autistic and whether they need to seek a more formal assessment. In either case, it is essential to highlight the possibility of high learning potential, if there is a suspicion that this could be part of a child's profile, and signpost and refer families for assessment.

When high learning potential is confirmed for a child who already has a diagnosis of autism, this could be the missing link in understanding how to help them further with the challenges they face and support them more specifically with regards to their strengths. In some cases, those who know the child best might suspect that the child was originally misdiagnosed as autistic as they learn more about the profiles and common behaviours of children with high learning potential.

When high learning potential is confirmed for a child who has not yet been diagnosed with autism, this may explain the child's particular strengths and challenges fully and a further diagnosis of autism does not need to be pursued. However, if the confirmation of high learning potential does not fully explain the child's challenges it may be that further assessment for autism is needed. However, the information already gained about the child's cognitive abilities will be beneficial to the autism assessment and diagnostic team.

Be sure to always approach the subject of further assessment for high learning potential and/or autism sensitively, and keep in mind that the reason is to understand a child's strengths and challenges better to help them more effectively. It should never cause more stress and confusion for the child, their parents or carers or other significant people in their life.

Differences

Being a "therapist on the ground" may make it hard to try and figure out whether a child has high learning potential, is autistic or both, especially in the absence of previous investigations done by other professionals. However, therapists may find it helpful to informally refer to the information provided in the High Learning Potential/Autism/DME Checklist (HADC) in Table 4.1. This is based on the Giftedness/Asperger's Disorder

Table 4.1 High Learning Potential/Autism/DME Checklist (HADC). Adapted from Amend et al (2008)

High Learning Potential / Autism / DME Checklist (HADC)
Based on Giftedness/Asperger's Disorder Checklist,
Amend, Beaver-Gavin, Schuler, and Beights (2008)
An individual with DME will present with characteristics from both columns.

High Learning Potential	Autism with unimpaired language and intelligence
Memory and Attention	
Excellent memory for facts and information about a variety of topics	Superb memory for facts and detailed information related to selected topics of special interest
Typically accurate recall of names of people and faces	Poor recall for names of people and faces
Dislikes rote memorisation tasks although he/she may do it well	Enjoys thinking about and remembering details, facts, and figures
Intense focus on topics of interest	Intense focus on primary topic of interest
If distracted, is likely to return to a task quickly with or without redirection	If distracted, redirecting to task may be difficult
Don't usually mind being distracted by others	Reacts negatively if concentration is broken by others
Speech and Language	
Communicates understanding of abstract ideas	Thinks and communicates in concrete and literal terms with less abstraction
Rich and interesting verbal style	Monotone verbal style
Engages others in interests	Style or content lacks reciprocity and engagement of others in their personal interests
Asks challenging questions that build on one another	Asks questions that are factual, basic and are disconnected
Expressive language/speech pattern of an older child	Speech has inappropriate formality in some situations
Elaborates with or without prompts	Little or no elaboration with run-on speech
Understands and engages in sophisticated and/or socially reciprocal humour, irony and sarcasm	Misunderstands jokes involving social reciprocity
Understands cause/effect or give and take conversation	Has difficulty understanding give and take of conversation
Able to communicate distress verbally	Communicates distress with actions rather than words
Social and Emotional	
Able to identify and name friends	May not be able to identify or name friends
Easily makes friends with people who share interests	Demonstrates significant difficulty and lacks understanding of how to establish and keep friends
Enjoys high social status in some circles	Unlikely to enjoy high social status
Aware of social norms	Indifferent to social norms of dress and behaviour
Keenly aware the he/she is different from peers	Limited recognition of differences with peers

(Continued)

Table 4.1 (Continued)

High Learning Potential / Autism / DME Checklist (HADC)
Based on Giftedness/Asperger's Disorder Checklist,
Amend, Beaver-Gavin, Schuler, and Beights (2008)
An individual with DME will present with characteristics from both columns.

High Learning Potential	Autism with unimpaired language and intelligence
• Spontaneous sharing of enjoyment, activities, interests or accomplishments	• Little or no interest in spontaneous sharing of enjoyment, activities, interests or accomplishments
• Engages with others in conversation	• Shows significant difficulty engaging others and reciprocating in conversation
• Aware of another's perspective and able to take and understand others' viewpoints	• When younger or male presenting, assume others share his/her personal views
• Follows unwritten rules of social interactions	• Unaware of social conventions or the reasons behind them
• Shows keen social insight and an intuitive nature	• Lacks social insight
• Aware of others' emotions and recognises others' feelings easily	• Limited recognition of others' emotions unless clearly demonstrated or told
• Able to read social situations and respond to social cues	• Misreads social situations and may not respond (or even know how to respond) to social cues
• Shows empathy for others and able to comfort a friend in need	• Needs to be told or clearly demonstrated to be able to respond empathically. May be unable to cope with others' distress
Behavioural	
• May passively resist but will often go along with change	• Actively or aggressively resists change; rigid
• Questions rules and structure but can still follow them*	• Adheres strictly to rules and needs structure*
• Stimming (e.g. hand or finger flapping, twisting or complex body movements) not present	• Stimming (e.g. hand or finger flapping, twisting or complex body movements) are present
• When problems arise, he/she is typically distressed by them	• When problems arise, parents or teachers are distressed by them while student may be unaware of distressing situation unless personally affected
Motor Skills	
• Well-coordinated	• Lacks age-appropriate coordination
• Interested in participating in team sports	• Avoids participating in team sports
• Demonstrates appropriate development of self-help skills	• Delayed acquisition of self-help skills

*This is different between the three groups: DME adhere to their own rules and want others to adhere to them too. They will strongly question rules that don't fit their internal structure.

Checklist (GADC) © Pre-Referral Checklist[14] but has been updated to include terminology used in the UK and to be more specific about some items. It can be used when a therapist observes a child during interactions with others who have similar intellectual abilities or interests as the child and from the therapist's observations of the child's insights about how others view them and their behaviours. Please note that the checklist is based on the research and clinical experience of the population by the authors of the original checklist and Andrea Anguera, doctoral researcher at the University of York and Senior Assessor at Potential Plus UK, but it has not been validated and norm-referenced. The checklist should therefore be used as a guide only, designed to facilitate appropriate interventions in the prereferral stage. It should not be used as a substitute for formal and comprehensive evaluation when further study is necessary to determine causes for behaviour.

A real-life example of a child where high learning potential and autism were suspected:

A few years ago one of the authors (Mariza) was asked to work with a seven-year-old child with handwriting difficulties. His teacher noted that his handwriting speed and volume was not consistent with his observed intelligence levels and verbal ability. They started working together on this goal, and his handwriting speed improved in the one-to-one therapy setting. However, this did not translate into his daily writing in the classroom, and on further investigation, his teacher reported that one of the main problems was that this child sometimes did not engage with the lessons. He rather seemed to daydream, and the teacher described him as being "away with the fairies". In test situations though, he focused very well and often got the best results for maths out of the whole class.

At the time, this child had an obsession with tractors. In fact, when first assessed, he told Mariza that one of his favourite tractors was a "combine harvester". She asked him to explain how it worked, and he started off with an intricate explanation of its mechanics, but then stopped halfway and said, "It's no use. It is too complicated, and you won't understand it anyway".

The child's school was situated on farmland, and the school itself had a few tractors for the ground staff to maintain the grounds. It transpired that the child was often listening out for the tractors in class at specific times of the day and subsequently thinking about tractors either before or after he heard them, which was often the reason for his daydreaming.

The child's teacher was very experienced and caring but became convinced the child was autistic. Mariza, on the other hand, thought he had high learning potential which was not yet confirmed or recognised, though she could not rule out the possibility of autism (even though it is not down to occupational therapists to diagnose in isolation). This was due to the fact that the child seemed to have limited insight into himself and his abilities, seemed very content with his own company, was not bothered if he was alone during playtime, happily went along with things and responded well to structured sessions.

When intervention with the child ended, the family had still not decided whether to proceed with assessments for either autism or high learning potential. They felt the child's needs and strengths were understood well enough by this time, by them and his teacher, to ensure both his needs and strengths were suitably catered for. Mariza felt the goal of highlighting the possibility that the child had high learning potential as an alternative to autism, or co-occurring with autism, was achieved.

Best therapy approach to help children with HLP who are also autistic

For a child with DME/2e who is autistic, as with any other child, therapy should be directed towards the areas of functional difficulty (or activity participation challenges) identified in the initial assessment and which the child, in partnership with their parents or carers, has chosen to work on. These may be related to the life spheres of personal care and self-management, work or school and leisure. This subsequently determines the therapy approach, or blend of therapy approaches, therapists will use.

When the child's functional difficulties relate to motor skills, such as handwriting or a teeth-brushing activity that may or may not include difficulties with the correct sequencing of the task, we have found top-down approaches such as the CO-OP or some of its principles and elements effective as part of an eclectic approach. We also find other occupational therapy techniques helpful. For example, backward chaining of activities, grading the difficulty level of activities, using visuals for the sequencing of tasks, providing equipment and/or environmental adaptations such as pencil grips and writing slopes are all effective. This is because these approaches all involve a strong cognitive element that children with DME/2e respond well to when introduced and explained. However, there are many times when incorporating a bottom-up approach is helpful, such as working on improving core body and hand muscle strength; although this will be decided in partnership with the child. An occupational therapist's personal style and preference may be purist in either a top-down or bottom-up approach. This is fine, as long as consideration is given to how cognitive elements can be brought into the therapy provision and the relationship with the child and their family or carers.

When the child's functional difficulties relate to sensory processing differences that specifically relate to sensory modulation or sensory processing patterns, such as being unable to cope in school with unexpected noises like the alarm bell going off, or noise levels in the class rising (see Chapter 5), and/or some of the non-OT factors we have described earlier in Chapter 4 such as perfectionism and an inflexible way of perceiving the motives of others affecting the ability to socialise and participate in leisure activities, we suggest using the DME-C approach that we present in this book.

As occupational therapists get to know a child in therapy sessions and monitor their progress, it will become clear whether occupational therapy on its own is sufficient to address the child's functional difficulties, or whether the child will benefit from further referral to an appropriate professional.

> **Consider this quote by Albert Einstein. It begs the question, "Was he just gifted, or perhaps also autistic"?**
>
> My passionate sense of social justice and social responsibility has always contrasted oddly with my pronounced lack of need for direct contact with other human beings and human communities. I am truly a "lone traveller" and have never belonged to my country, my home, my friends, or even my immediate family, with my whole heart…
>
> (Einstein, *The World as I See It*)

Attention Deficit Hyperactivity Disorder or ADHD

Definition

ADHD[15,16] is a neurodevelopmental disorder that affects approximately 5 to 8% of school aged children and is a lifelong condition. It is characterised by a persistent pattern of inattention and or hyperactivity and impulsivity, which affect a person's functioning, development and learning.

ADHD makes focussing on everyday requests and routines challenging and affects all the spheres of a person's life: personal care and self-management, work or school and leisure activities, including friendships. Children with ADHD can be defiant, socially inept or aggressive and present predominantly with inattentiveness, hyperactivity-impulsivity or a combined presentation.

When children with ADHD have a predominant presentation of inattentiveness, they often fail to give close attention to detail, or they make careless mistakes in schoolwork or during other activities. They have difficulty sustaining their attention in tasks or play activities or are easily distracted, do not seem to listen when spoken to directly, often do not follow through on instructions and fail to finish schoolwork or chores. These children have difficulties with organising tasks and activities, avoid or dislike tasks that require sustained mental effort such as homework, often lose things necessary for activities such as pencils and books and are often forgetful in daily activities. These children are sometimes only identified later in childhood.

When children with ADHD have a predominant presentation of hyperactivity-impulsivity, they often fidget with or tap their hands and feet or squirm in their seats and cannot sit still for long e.g. in class. They are unable to play or engage in leisure activities quietly and are often "on the go", which others may experience as restlessness or have difficulties keeping up with. Younger children may run around or climb inappropriately whilst older children may appear restless. These children may talk excessively, blurt out an answer in class before the teacher has completed asking a question, struggle with turn-taking in conversations and interrupt others, have difficulty waiting their turn such as when standing in a line and intrude on others such as starting to use people's things without asking or getting permission. These children are often identified earlier on in childhood than those with ADHD who present with inattentiveness only.

ADHD is formally recognised by international organisations including the World Health Organisation. The full criteria for the diagnosis of ADHD is listed in the *Diagnostic and Statistical Manual of Mental Disorders, Fifth Edition* (DSM-V) and the *International Statistical Classification of Diseases and Related Health Problems* (ICD-11).

High learning potential and ADHD

Occupational therapists can familiarise themselves with what ADHD is, and how it presents in children, by visiting websites such as American Psychological Association https://www.apa.org/topics/adhd and doing training courses on the topic specifically designed for occupational therapists. This is worthwhile because, similar to autism, there are many similarities between ADHD and high learning potential, which can lead to children with the latter being misdiagnosed with ADHD. However, it is possible for children to have both ADHD and high learning potential, in which case they have the profile of DME/2e. In fact, it is estimated that 10% of children with ADHD also have high learning potential/are gifted.[17] Of course, both these groups of children often have additional challenges such as sensory processing differences.

Similarities

Some examples of traits that are similar in children with ADHD and children with high learning potential are that both often display high activity levels, difficulties paying attention, impulsivity, daydreaming[18] and a need for cognitive stimulation. However, the reason that children with ADHD display these behaviours can be found in the current thinking as to the possible causes for ADHD. Among these is that ADHD is associated with an "underactive" frontal lobe and a hypoaroused brain state which may be responsible for gross motor hyperactivity and variable sustained attention.[19] In contrast, the reason that children with high learning potential display these behaviours can be explained by asynchronous development,[20] boredom in the classroom[21,22] or overexcitabilities,[23] specifically psychomotor, sensual and imaginational overexcitabilities.[24]

Whilst it may seem counterintuitive, both children with ADHD and those with high learning potential have the ability to hyperfocus on tasks for extended periods of time. However, children with high learning potential will generally be able to switch between tasks more easily than those with ADHD. Interestingly, a study[25] to compare how boys with DME/2e (specifically high learning potential and ADHD) and those with ADHD responded to the ability to shift between tasks, showed that the DME boys had more difficulty doing this than those with ADHD only. The researchers concluded this was because of the tendency of boys with DME/2e to maintain intense focus on tasks involving higher-level thinking skills, which is often seen as a strength and not a difficulty, but can clearly make switching between tasks more difficult.

For clarification, a child can have ADHD on its own, high learning potential on its own, or the two together, in which case they have the profile of DME/2e. However, a child with high learning potential can also be misdiagnosed with ADHD if the professionals in the assessment and diagnostic team have not assessed or considered the child's cognitive abilities and that certain behaviours overlap between ADHD and high learning potential.

Regardless of the setting paediatric occupational therapists work in, they should speak up if it is suspected that a child they are working with has high learning potential, whether that child already has a diagnosis of ADHD or not.

When a child already has a diagnosis of ADHD and high learning potential is later confirmed, it could help the child, their family and teachers understand the child's strengths and challenges better. This in turn can contribute to the child receiving better support to develop their high learning potential, alongside accommodations for their ADHD. As with autism, in some cases, the child's parents or carers might suspect that the child was originally misdiagnosed with ADHD as they learn more about the profiles and common behaviours of children with high learning potential.

If high learning potential is confirmed for a child who has not yet been diagnosed with ADHD, it may explain the child's particular strengths and challenges fully and a further diagnosis of ADHD does not need to be pursued. However, it may be that high learning potential does not explain all their challenges, and so further assessment for ADHD is needed. The information already gained regarding the child's cognitive abilities will be beneficial to the ADHD assessment and diagnostic team.

As always, please approach the subject of further assessment for high learning potential and or ADHD sensitively, and keep in mind that the reason is to understand a child's strengths and challenges better to help them more effectively. It should never cause more stress and confusion for the child, their parents or carers, or other significant people in their life.

Differences between children with both high learning potential and ADHD and those with high learning potential only

In literature, there seem to be few research articles available on the differences between children with "pure" ADHD versus "pure" high learning potential or giftedness. Rather, there seems to be more information on the differences between children with the DME/2e profile of high learning potential together with ADHD and those children who have high learning potential only.

In general, children with high learning potential and ADHD struggle more than their peers who have high learning potential without ADHD, in the following areas:

- Executive functioning skills, which specifically affects the child's ability to manage their own emotions and behaviours[26]

- Social and emotional problems, specifically immaturity, irresponsible behaviour and annoying behaviour[27]
- Low self-esteem, self-concept and overall happiness[28]
- Depression, generalised and separation anxiety disorder, social phobias and conduct disorder[29]
- Underachieving academically, avoiding homework, and difficulty initiating and staying on task[30]

Surprisingly, children with high learning potential and ADHD are thought to demonstrate more creative ability than children with high learning potential only.[31]

Best therapy approach to help children with HLP who also have ADHD

Following an assessment of a child with the DME/2e profile of high learning potential and ADHD, therapists may find that there are quite a lot of goals they and the child can work on together to address the participation challenges they have in various spheres of their life. These may include personal care, self-management, school and leisure, including socialising with friends. This could potentially mean longer-term involvement with the child. As always, our advice would be to focus on the areas that cause the child, their family and perhaps their teachers the most distress.

Often the main area of concern relates to the child's inability to sit still and focus on what their parents or teachers are saying or trying to teach them, particularly when it comes to doing tasks independently. Hand in hand with that, by the time the child gets to occupational therapy for help, it is quite possible they have developed low self-esteem due to feeling constantly misunderstood by others and/or efforts to be focussed not being successful. A mistrust of professionals and an inflexible way of perceiving the motives of others often follows closely behind.

A poem by a child with DME/2e, who has high learning potential, ADHD and sensory processing differences. Used with permission from the child and his parents:

> This Is Me
> Hi. My name is Jack. I am ten. I'm like you. I have hobbies.
> I play sports and video games, except for one thing: ADHD.
> It means I can't concentrate, which makes me impulsive and loud.
> It means I can't stop as easily as others.
> Sometimes, I make sounds without knowing.
> It makes me sad when people who don't understand shout at me.
> It makes me feel lonely, down and alienated.
> It's really upsetting.
> I wish more people knew!

First of all, it is important to determine whether the child's behaviour, which appears as sensory seeking, is due to ADHD, sensory processing differences, intellectual boredom or a combination of these. Often the best way to do this, although not fail-safe, is by the process of elimination. For instance, is the child less fidgety and more able to focus when they have taken their ADHD medication? If this is the case, then you know ADHD plays a part. If the child is very "on the go" despite having taken the correct dose of ADHD medication, then there is a sensory element. If the child is noticeably more engaged with academic work that is more challenging and/or presented in more depth, then intellectual boredom plays a part.

Occupational therapists may be working with a child where the family has opted for the child not to take any ADHD medication. This may initially make it more difficult to identify the reason for a child's behaviour, although it is our experience that with time and as a therapist works with the child, the reasons will become clearer to the therapist. For one, if "on the go" behaviour is mainly a result of a child's ADHD, then sensory based interventions on their own will have very little effect.

In general, children with ADHD and sensory processing differences benefit most from occupational therapy that is multifaceted.[32] For example, intervention should consist of a combination of behavioural management strategies, sensory based strategies such as participation in sensory diets and the provision of equipment such as fiddle toys, adapting the physical environment and parent/teacher training.

In our experience, children with high learning potential, ADHD, sensory processing differences, and difficulties with socialising and participating in leisure activities because of a combination of these factors and some of the non-OT factors (perfectionism and a fixed mindset) respond well to the DME-C approach. This is because the DME-C approach in itself is a multifaceted approach. However, occupational therapists need to ensure they specifically include simple strategies to encourage the child to stay on task, such as verbally commending and praising effort and desired behaviours the moment they are observed. When a therapist acknowledges they can see a child is trying, it will help the child to understand the therapist is not expecting them to do things perfectly, get things right and/or have textbook behaviour all the time.

If a child continues to struggle to stay on task in sessions, but is highly motivated to work on the goals which have been set together at the start of therapy, then a therapeutic contract can be considered which sets out the desired behaviours in sessions to reach the goals. Such a therapeutic contract should only be drawn up in collaboration with the child if the child feels it will help them, and then signed by the child and therapist. Please note that the child should understand the reason for the contract, and if they are not able to keep to its terms, the way forward should be discussed with the child. See Figure 4.1 for an example of a therapy contract that has been used successfully.

The therapist and child can also agree on using some other motivators to help the child stay on task in sessions. For example, the child can choose an activity or game they would like to play at the end of a session to motivate them to complete the necessary session aims in

Figure 4.1 Example of basic therapy contract.

Child's therapy contract:
I commit to the following responsibilities expected of me during and between therapy sessions:

- I will do my best to focus my brain on the topics we are discussing in sessions and not try to distract the therapist.
- I will do the occupational therapy homework tasks each week and bring it along to the next session in a folder.
- I will do three or four sensory diet activities each day before I go to school.

the allocated time. Giving the child a certificate of completion once they have finished their occupational therapy program is often a welcome surprise (and motivator to continue using the strategies learnt during sessions!).

Conclusion

We trust that occupational therapists now have a clearer understanding of their vital role in helping all children with DME/2e, and that they will use the information we have shared in Chapter 4 as a springboard to further research ways in which to complement their therapy provision for children with DME/2e. In Chapter 5, we will have a more thorough discussion on sensory processing differences and DME/2e. We will also start bridging the gap between the occupational therapy and gifted/high learning potential communities by explaining how sensory-related terminology correlates with Dabrowski's overexcitabilities, particularly sensual and psychomotor overexcitabilities. This will be an important starting point for therapists when working with this neurodivergent group of children before diving deeper into the DME-C approach.

Notes

* The authors note autistic spectrum condition or autism are the preferred current terms. We have used autistic spectrum disorder here as this is what is used in diagnostic and health guidelines.

References

1 Adapted from: Yates, D., & Boddison, A. (2020) *The School Handbook for Dual and Multiple Exceptionality; High Learning Potential with Special Educational Needs or Disabilities*. Routledge.
2 Silverman, L. K., & Waters, J. L. (1988, November). *The Silverman/Waters Checklist: A new culture-fair identification instrument*. National Association for Gifted Children 35th Annual Convention, Orlando, FL.
3 Derived (and further expanded) from websites:
  - CanChild (n.d.) *Developmental Coordination Disorder*. CanChild Diagnoses. Retrieved July 7, 2022, from https://canchild.ca/en/diagnoses/developmental-coordination-disorder.
  - Movement Matters (n.d.) *Frequently Asked Questions*. Movement Matters. Retrieved July 7, 2022, from http://www.movementmattersuk.org/dcd-dyspraxia-adhd-spld/developmental-disorders-documentation/frequently-asked-questions.aspx.

- Dyspraxia Foundation (n.d.) *Diagnosis*. What is Dyspraxia? Retrieved July 7, 2022, from https://dyspraxiafoundation.org.uk/what_is_dyspraxia/diagnosis/.
4. Derived from websites:
   - Dyspraxia Foundation (n.d.) *Diagnosis*. What is Dyspraxia? Retrieved July 7, 2022, from https://dyspraxiafoundation.org.uk/what_is_dyspraxia/diagnosis/.
   - Star Institute (n.d.) *Subtypes of SPD*. What is SPD? Retrieved July 7, 2022, from https://sensoryhealth.org/basic/subtypes-of-spd.
5. Miller J. L., Nielson M. D., Schoen A. S. (2012). Attention deficit hyperactivity disorder and sensory modulation disorder: a comparison of behavior and physiology. Res. Dev. Disabil. 33, 804–818 10.1016/j.ridd.2011.12.005
6. Fried W. Dyspraxia and DCD: An Overview. Retrieved July 21, 2022, from https://www.smartkidswithld.org/first-steps/what-are-learning-disabilities/dyspraxia-dcd-overview/.
7. Vaivre-Douret, L., Hamdioui, S. & Cannafarina, A. (2020) *The Influence of IQ Levels on Clinical Features of Developmental Coordination Disorder*. Journal of Psychiatry and Psychiatric Disorders 4. 218-234. Retrieved July 22, 2022, from https://www.fortune-journals.com/articles/the-influence-of-iq-levels-on-clinical-features-of-developmental-coordination-disorder.html.
8. Haase, J. & Sheard, W. (2019, December 5) *RCCX Theory and Giftedness: A Promising New Line of Research*. GroGifted. https://www.gro-gifted.org/rccx-theory-and-giftedness-a-promising-new-line-of-research/.
9. ICAN (n.d.) *The COOP Approach*. ICANCOOP. Retrieved July 7, 2022, from https://ican-coop.org/pages/the-co-op-approach.
10. National Autistic Society (n.d.) What is Autism? Advice and Guidance. Retrieved July 7, 2022, from https://www.autism.org.uk/advice-and-guidance/what-is-autism.
11. World Health Organisation (2022, March 30) *Autism* [Fact Sheet]. https://www.who.int/news-room/fact-sheets/detail/autism-spectrum-disorders.
12. National Institute for Health and Care Excellence (2012, updated 2021) *Autism Spectrum Disorder in Adults: Diagnosis and Management* [NICE Guideline CG142]. https://www.nice.org.uk/guidance/cg142/chapter.
13. Asperger Syndrome (2022, June 25) In *Wikipedia*. https://en.wikipedia.org/wiki/Asperger_syndrome.
14. Amend, E. R., Beaver-Gavin, K., Schuler, P., Beights, R. (2008). Giftedness/Asperger's Disorder Checklist (GADC) Pre-Referral Checklist.
15. Derived from:
    - American Psychiatric Association (2013). *ADHD: attention deficit and hyperactivity disorder*. In *Diagnostic and statistical manual of mental disorders (5th ed.)*.
    - American Psychological Association (n.d.) *ADHD*. Retrieved July 8, 2022, from https://www.apa.org/topics/adhd.
16. World Health Organisation (2019) *Attention Deficit Hyperactivity Disorder (ADHD)* [Fact Sheet]. https://applications.emro.who.int/docs/EMRPUB_leaflet_2019_mnh_214_en.pdf?ua=1&ua=1.
17. Antshel, Kevin. (2008). *Attention-Deficit Hyperactivity Disorder in the context of a high intellectual quotient/giftedness*. Developmental disabilities research reviews. 14. 293-9. 10.1002/ddrr.34.
    Chae, P.K. & Kim, J.-H & Noh, Kwonkuk. (2003). *Diagnosis of ADHD among gifted children in relation to KEDI-WISC and T.O.V.A. performance*. Gifted Child Quarterly. 47. 192-201.
18. Hartnett, D. & Nelson, Jason & Rinn, Anne. (2004). *Gifted or ADHD? The possibility of misdiagnosis*. Roeper Review. 26. 73-76. 10.1080/02783190409554245.
19. Loo, S.K., Hale, T.S., Macion, J., Hanada, G., McGough, J.J., McCracken, J.T., Smalley, S.L. (2009). *Cortical activity patterns in ADHD during arousal, activation and sustained attention*. Neuropsychologia. 2009 Aug;47(10):2114-9.
20. Silverman, L.. (1997). *The Construct of Asynchronous Development*. Peabody Journal of Education., 72(3), 36-58. https://doi.org/info:doi/
21. Gallagher, J., Harradine, C. C., & Coleman, M. R. (1997). *Challenge or boredom? Gifted students' views on their schooling*. Roeper Review: A Journal on Gifted Education, 19(3), 132-141. https://doi.org/10.1080/02783199709553808.

22. Webb, J. T., & Latimer, D. (1993). *ERIC Digest ADHD and Children Who are Gifted.* Exceptional Children, 60(2), 183-184. https://doi.org/10.1177/001440299306000213.
23. Dabrowski, K. (1964). *Positive disintegration.* Little, Brown.
    Mendaglio, S. (2012). *Overexcitabilities and Giftedness Research A Call for a Paradigm Shift.* Journal for the Education of the Gifted. 35. 207-219. 10.1177/0162353212451704.
24. Rinn, A. N. & Reynolds, M. J. (2012) *Overexcitabilities and ADHD in the Gifted: An Examination*, Roeper Review, 34:1, 38-45, DOI: 10.1080/02783193.2012.627551.
25. Kalbfleisch, M. L. (2001). *Electroencephalographic (EEG) differences between boys with average and high-aptitude with and without attention deficit hyperactivity disorder (ADHD) during task transitions.* Dissertation Abstracts International: Section B. Sciences and Engineering,62(1-B), 96.
26. Brown, K.W., West, A.M., Loverich, T.M., Biegel, G.M. (2011). Assessing adolescent mindfulness: validation of an adapted Mindful Attention Awareness Scale in adolescent normative and psychiatric populations. *Psychological Assessment.* doi:10.1037/a0021338.
27. Moon, S., Zentall, S., Grskovic, J., Hall, A. & Stormont, M. (2001). *Emotional and Social Characteristics of Boys with AD/HD and Giftedness: A Comparative Case Study.* Journal for the Education of the Gifted. 24. 10.1177/016235320102400302.
28. Foley-Nicpon, M., Rickels, H., Assouline, S. & Richards, A. (2012). *Self-Esteem and Self-Concept Examination Among Gifted Students With ADHD.* Journal for the Education of the Gifted. 35. 220-240. 10.1177/0162353212451735.
29. Antshel, K. M., Faraone, S. V., Fremont, W., Monuteaux, M. C., Kates, W. R., Doyle, A., Mick, E., & Biederman, J. (2007). Comparing ADHD in Velocardiofacial Syndrome to Idiopathic ADHD: A Preliminary Study. *Journal of Attention Disorders*, 11(1), 64-73. https://doi.org/10.1177/1087054707299397
30. Zentall, S., Moon, S., Hall, A. & Grskovic, J. (2001). *Learning and Motivational Characteristics of Boys With AD/HD and/or Giftedness.* Exceptional Children. 67. 499-519. 10.1177/001440290106700405.
31. Fugate, C., Zentall, S. & Gentry, M. (2013). *Creativity and Working Memory in Gifted Students With and Without Characteristics of Attention Deficit Hyperactive Disorder: Lifting the Mask.* Gifted Child Quarterly. 57. 234-246. 10.1177/0016986213500069.
32. Chu, S. (2003). *Attention deficit hyperactivity disorder (ADHD) part one: a review of the literature.* British Journal of Therapy and Rehabilitation, 10(5), 218-227.
    Chu, S., & Reynolds, F. (2007). *Occupational Therapy for Children with Attention Deficit Hyperactivity Disorder (ADHD), Part 1: A Delineation Model of Practice.* British Journal of Occupational Therapy, 70(9), 372-383. https://doi.org/10.1177/030802260707000902.

Chapter five
DME/Twice Exceptionality and Sensory Processing Differences

Introduction

Sensory processing difficulties or differences are probably one of the most widely discussed topics in occupational therapy. It both unites and divides professionals, which we are not here to do. Our main concern is to confirm the fact that children with HLP or giftedness can have sensory processing differences, which can have a significant impact on their lives if not addressed appropriately and in a timely manner. We have worked and continue to work on the ground with children with DME/2e and see the positive change that occupational therapy brings.

In this chapter, we share the literature base for sensory processing differences we use, which is the Sensory Processing Disorder Model by Dr Lucy Miller and the Model of Sensory Processing by Prof Winnie Dunn. We acknowledge that there are other models which provide alternative explanations and terminology for sensory processing differences, such as *Sensory Integration: Theory and Practice, Third Edition* by Anita C. Bundy and Shelly J. Lane. Therapists can continue to use whichever model they are familiar with and are able to explain to the children with DME/2e they work with. Furthermore, in Chapter 5 we will discuss how sensory processing differences relate to HLP and how some of its terminology correlates with Dabrowski's overexcitabilities which were introduced in Chapter 2.

Sensory Processing Differences

Definition

Sensory integration, or SI,[1] is the neurological process by which the brain registers, interprets and organises sensory messages received through the senses from the environment and/or from within the body, in order to have appropriate motor and/or behavioural responses so a person can successfully interact with their environment.

The theory of sensory integration was first formulated by Dr Anna Jean Ayres in the 1970s and early 1980s. She was an occupational therapist, educational psychologist and neuroscientist who did extensive research into sensory integration and associated difficulties, through her work with children with learning disabilities. In Dr Ayres's own words,[2] "SI is the neurological process that organises sensations from one's own body and from the environment and makes it possible to use the body effectively with the environment".

Difficulties with sensory integration, in other words when the brain has difficulty registering, interpreting and organising sensory messages received through the senses from the

DOI: 10.4324/9781003334033-5

environment and/or from within the body, result in inappropriate motor and/or behavioural responses, meaning the child struggles to successfully interact with their environment. **These difficulties are described by an array of terms with roughly the same meaning and they may be used interchangeably by various professionals.** This is because to date there is not one definitive and recognised term to describe difficulties with sensory integration. The terms that are or were used are:

- Sensory processing disorder or SPD;[3] probably one of the most well known and recognised terms in the world
- Sensory processing difficulties;[4] also very well known and preferred by many professionals due to the fact that SPD is not recognised as an independent diagnosis in the *Diagnostic and Statistical Manual of Mental Disorders 5* or DSM-V (American Psychiatric Association 2013) and therefore using the term SPD should be avoided
- Sensory processing differences; a term currently gaining popularity because it demedicalises the term and acknowledges it as a neurodivergence
- Sensory regulation dysfunction, sensory integration dysfunction or sensory dysfunction disorder;[5] some older terms

For the reasons stated above and due to personal preference, we choose to use the terms sensory processing differences or difficulties in this book, interchangeably.

Whilst SPD is not an independent condition listed in the DSM-V, it is a diagnostic entity in the *Diagnostic Classification of Mental Health and Developmental Disorders of Infancy and Early Childhood-Revised Manual* (generally known as Zero to Three),[6] and in the *Interdisciplinary Council on Developmental and Learning Disorders Diagnostic Manual for Infants and Young Children* (ICDL-DMIC).[7]

Importantly, sensory processing differences often form part of the diagnostic criteria for other disorders in the DSM-V, such as autism spectrum disorder. This inadvertently confirms its existence and importance as a set of difficulties that can negatively impact on a child's learning, coordination, behaviour, language or sensorimotor development, which in turn impacts on their ability to successfully participate in activities of daily living.[8] In other words, it can affect all the spheres of a child's life: personal care and self-management, work, school and leisure activities including friendships. It may cause children poor attention, stress, anxiety and even depression.

Before we look at the types of sensory processing differences a child can have, let us briefly review the eight sensory systems in the human body, including their main functions with regards to sensory processing. We have summarised this in Figure 5.1. Please note this is an overview only, and we highly recommend occupational therapists do further research, study or training into the sensory systems of the human body as part of their professional development journey.

To recap, when the body's nervous system accurately registers, interprets and organises sensory messages or stimuli, and a person is able to filter out irrelevant stimuli and concentrate on relevant stimuli, we have adequate sensory processing, or what Dr Ayres described as a "free flowing traffic system" in the brain. However, if the nervous system processes and responds

Figure 5.1 The sensory systems.

Senses that register sensory information from the external environment

Sensory system	Sensory receptors	Main functions
Visual	Vision receptors, or retina containing rods and cones (photoreceptors), at the back of the eyes	**Seeing** Visual sensory processing is the ability to correctly focus on a person or object relevant at a particular time, whilst not giving attention to other visual images, and having an appropriate action in response. It also contributes to good visual perceptual abilities and postural control
Auditory	Auditory receptors, or hair cells found in the organ of Corti situated in the cochlea in the inner ear	**Hearing** Auditory sensory processing is the ability to correctly register relevant sound waves from the environment through the ears (hearing), whilst not giving attention to background noise, and having an appropriate action in response. Good auditory sensory processing is fundamental to speech and language development, communication, understanding instructions, reading, writing and timing movements
Olfactory	Olfactory receptors, located in the olfactory epithelium in the nose	**Smelling and tasting** Olfactory sensory processing is the ability to correctly register smell through the nose, and gustatory sensory processing is the ability to correctly register taste through the mouth in order to have an appropriate action in response. These two sensory systems work closely together. Being able to eat and drink a variety of foods and drinks and not have an aversive reaction to its particular smell, taste or texture allows a child the opportunity to have a healthy diet.
Gustatory	Taste receptors; or papillae containing taste buds, mainly on the tongue in the mouth	
Tactile	Tactile receptors, or tactile mechanoreceptors, located in the skin	**Perceiving touch** The skin detects external temperature, pain and light touch. The main functions of the tactile sensory system are: 1. Protection, through a heightened awareness that the child may be in contact with something dangerous or threatening. Linked to survival behaviours such as fight, flight and freeze 2. Discrimination, to help a child determine what they are touching or what is touching them 3. Contributes to regulating alertness levels or "how awake you feel" 4. Contributes to overall child development, including social and emotional stability

(Continued)

Figure 5.1 (Continued)

Senses that register sensory information from within the body		
Sensory system	Sensory receptors	Main functions
Vestibular	Vestibular system in the inner ear	**Sensing movement and balance** The vestibular sensory system is activated by gravity and static and dynamic movements, or in other words, by movements of the head (in relation to gravity) in different directions and whether a person is standing still or moving – and, when moving, how fast they are moving and in which direction. Vestibular sensory processing occurs on a subconscious level. The main functions of the vestibular sensory system are: 1. Movement 2. Balance 3. Correctly perceiving the sensation of gravity 4. Contributes to head control and a stable visual field "to see clearly whilst moving" 5. Contributes to regulating muscle tone and body posture in order to participate in tasks, e.g. sitting to write 6. Contributes to coordinating the two sides of the body for activities, such as tying shoelaces 7. Contributes to regulating alertness levels or "how awake you feel" 8. Contributes to spatial awareness By processing vestibular information correctly, a child feels secure during movement, which helps them to develop both physical and emotional core stability.
Proprioceptive	Skeletal muscles, joints, ligaments and tendons	**Sensing body position and muscle control** The proprioceptive sensory system is activated by pressure on and pulling of the skeletal muscles, joints, ligaments and tendons. Proprioceptive sensory processing can occur on a conscious level, e.g. being able to purposefully press harder or softer with a pencil when writing. It also occurs on an unconscious level, such as the knee reflex, which is automatically activated by tapping on the patellar ligament. The main functions of the proprioceptive sensory system are: 1. Body position or spatial awareness, described as "knowing where you are in space without needing to look"

(Continued)

Figure 5.1 (Continued)

Senses that register sensory information from within the body		
Sensory system	Sensory receptors	Main functions
		2. Applying the correct amount of muscle force when handling objects, described as "knowing how hard to handle objects"
		3. Applying the correct amount of muscle force when moving, which will differ depending on the activity, e.g. walking vs. running
		4. Contributes to regulating muscle tone and body posture in order to participate in tasks, e.g. sitting to write
		5. Contributes to coordinating the two sides of the body for activities, such as tying shoelaces
		6. Contributes to regulating alertness levels or "how awake you feel"
		7. Contributes to feeling calm and regulated
Interoception	Various internal organs detected by receptors in our internal organs	**Sensing basic functions or physical conditions of the body, also involved in emotional regulation**
		Examples include:
		1. Hunger, thirst, bladder feeling full
		2. Anger, embarrassment, happiness, fear
		Also contributes to the ability to appropriately self-regulate

to incoming sensory messages inappropriately, it is like having a "traffic jam" in the brain. The child is not able to respond as they, or others, would expect them to. This could have a detrimental effect on their ability to participate in relevant everyday activities, and in this case, we refer to the child having **sensory processing differences or difficulties**.

As mentioned in the introduction to this chapter, we draw on the Sensory Processing Disorder Model by Dr Lucy Miller (SPD) and the Model of Sensory Processing by Prof Winnie Dunn to describe sensory processing differences, but we tend to use terminology from both models interchangeably. This is to accommodate the understanding of a wider range of parents and children who may have been exposed to either model.

Important

The SPD subcategory "sensory modulation disorder" by Dr Lucy Miller, and "sensory processing patterns" as defined by Prof. Winnie Dunn (see explanations below), are the main categories of sensory processing differences that we address in the DME-C therapy approach. However, we will highlight our recommendations for addressing the

SPD subcategories "sensory based motor disorders" and "sensory based discrimination disorders" at the end of this chapter, under the heading "Best therapy approach to help children with HLP who also have sensory processing differences".

The Sensory Processing Disorder Model[9] proposes there are three main subtypes of sensory processing differences. A child can have difficulties in only one of these areas, or across various of these areas. Every child is different, so the way one child presents can differ greatly from another. The three main subtypes are:

1. Sensory modulation disorder
2. Sensory based motor disorder
3. Sensory discrimination disorder

Sensory Modulation Disorder

Sensory modulation disorder is when a child has difficulty regulating their responses to incoming sensory messages. This is when a child over- or under-responds to stimuli, or excessively seeks out more stimuli. Children often have a mixed sensory profile of these sensory based behaviours, not just across the sensory systems but also in the same sensory system. For example, a child can be sensory seeking with regards to movement (vestibular) but sensory avoiding with regards to touch (tactile); or a child can be both over responsive to and seek out touch experiences (tactile), and be over responsive to noise (auditory). Whatever a child's profile, they struggle to feel "just right" or regulated in order to participate in the task at hand.

When a child over responds to sensory stimuli, it means they are more sensitive to those particular stimuli than other people. The child perceives "normal" sensation as harmful and has a "fight, flight or freeze response" when presented with the stimuli. Typical examples are when a child pulls away when being touched (avoiding), covers their ears in noisy environments (avoiding), becomes aggressive in visually busy places (fight) or has a meltdown when eating certain foods (avoiding, fight, flight).

When a child under responds to sensory stimuli, it means they are less aware of sensations than other people, and they typically need more and a higher intensity of the stimuli before they will respond. For instance, they may only register that a teacher has called them on the third or fourth repetition. Under responders are generally passive and their sensory processing differences often go unnoticed because they do not cause any trouble. Furthermore, they have poor body awareness and difficulty coordinating motor tasks, and they may not be aware of pain following an injury such as may be caused by falling over.

When a child noticeably seeks out more of a particular stimulus than those around them, we say they are sensory seekers or cravers, or what we refer to as the "jumping off the wall, fiddly, in your face and in your space kids". They are constantly on the go, need to touch others and objects constantly, like crashing and bumping into people and things, prefer music or television turned up loudly or like bright and/or flashing lights. However, whilst getting more stimulation can help, these children often get over stimulated and may not become calmer and more regulated.

Sensory modulation disorder and sensory processing patterns

In the Model of Sensory Processing[10] Prof Dunn uses the term "sensory processing patterns more or less than others" to describe sensory processing differences. It is based on the two constructs of neurological thresholds (how quickly the nervous system responds to stimuli) and self-regulation (how the child deals with the stimuli).

Regarding neurological thresholds, a child can either have a low neurological threshold where the nervous system is easily activated or a high neurological threshold where the nervous system takes longer to be activated. With regards to self-regulation, the child may either respond passively to the incoming stimuli, such as allowing it to happen before responding, if at all, or the child may respond actively to incoming stimuli, such as trying to get away from or control the stimuli they may encounter in everyday life. When the neurological threshold and self-regulation continua interact with each other, they create the four sensory processing patterns of registration/bystander, sensitivity/sensor, seeking/seeker and avoiding/avoider. Please see Figure 5.2.

For clarification, seeking refers to the degree to which a child obtains sensory input, avoiding refers to the degree to which a child is bothered by sensory input, sensitivity refers to the degree to which a child detects sensory input and registration refers to the degree to which a child misses sensory input. However, Prof Dunn proposes that a child's sensory processing patterns only need to be addressed if they have reported activity participation challenges, such as moving so excessively in class that they are unable to follow the teacher's instructions.

When working with children with DME/2e who have sensory processing differences which relate to sensory modulation or sensory processing patterns, occupational therapists may prefer to use terminology from both models interchangeably, as we tend to do, or they may prefer to strictly use terminology from only one model. Whatever the choice, the child and family should understand what is meant, not only for themselves, but also when they speak and advocate for themselves with others. This also relates to writing formal occupational therapy reports, and we suggest a glossary is included with a summary of the terms used.

Figure 5.2 Dunn's four sensory patterns.

Neurological threshold	Self-regulation	
	PASSIVE	**ACTIVE**
HIGH	Registration/Bystander	Seeking/Seeker
LOW	Sensitivity/Sensor	Avoiding/Avoider

Figure 5.3 Correlation between terminology from Miller's and Dunn's models.

Miller's Sensory Processing Disorder Model	Dunn's Model of Sensory Processing
Under responder	Registration/Bystander
Over responder	Sensitivity/Sensor and Avoiding/Avoider
Sensory seeker	Seeking/Seeker

When using terms from both models we have just discussed, it may help to think of the informal correlation between terms which we have summarised in Figure 5.3.

High Learning Potential and Sensory Processing Differences

A study by the Star Institute[11] in the USA estimates that up to a **third** of children in the high learning potential/gifted community exhibit symptoms of sensory processing differences, which is significantly more than the 5% that pilot studies found in the general population. The most common form of sensory processing differences children with DME/2e display is a heightened awareness of and response to sensory stimulation[12] (sensory over responsiveness), but sensory seeking behaviour and sensory under responsiveness are also common in this group. Many children with DME/2e also have dyspraxia which is a type of sensory based motor disorder when viewed through the lens of the Sensory Processing Disorder Model[13] (see sensory based motor disorders in the next section), or developmental coordination disorder when viewed as a standalone motor skills disorder, as we discussed in Chapter 4 under the heading of developmental coordination disorder/DCD.

Our own observations from working with children with DME/2e and sensory processing differences are in line with these findings, with over responsiveness to auditory sensory stimuli and an increased and intense need for physical movement more than their peers being the most common reasons children and their parents/carers seek occupational therapy.

Sensory processing differences and Dabrowski's overexcitabilities

When parents of children with DME/2e who already know about their child's high learning potential approach occupational therapists for help, they will often use the term "overexcitabilities" to describe some of the associated challenges their child is experiencing. They have likely researched possible reasons for the difficulties and discussed these with others in a similar situation where they would have come across Dabrowski's overexcitabilities,[14] which we discussed in detail in Chapter 2. As a reminder, Dabrowski identified five areas in which children with high learning potential exhibit intense behaviours or overexcitabilities. These super-sensitivities fall into the categories of:

- Psychomotor, which is defined as high levels of energy
- Sensual, which relates to a heightened awareness of sensations

- Emotional, which relates to exceptional emotional sensitivity and often mental health problems
- Intellectual, which relates to a seemingly unquenchable thirst for knowledge
- Imaginational, which relates to vivid imaginations, causing them to often visualise the worst possibility in any situation

When occupational therapists are first confronted with the terms used in Dabrowski's overexcitabilities, it can seem daunting and confusing. However, on closer examination, some of the overexcitability terms correlate with the terms used to describe sensory processing differences which relate to sensory modulation or sensory processing patterns. This is because they are similar to how a child responds to incoming sensory stimuli. Understanding these similarities will go a long way in helping occupational therapists make sense of a child's difficulties in line with occupational therapy training. Furthermore, explaining these similarities or correlations to the children and parents will help them fit new terminology into their existing knowledge framework and empower them to be more effective advocates for their children.

Sensual overexcitabilities[15] mean a heightened awareness of the external five senses of vision, hearing, smell, taste and touch. However, the term does not differentiate between being sensory over responsive (sensitive/avoiding) or sensory seeking. It is therefore an umbrella term to describe being both over stimulated by sensory stimuli as well as seeking certain sensory stimuli. In our experience, children with DME/2e generally avoid sound, visually busy environments and touch experiences, but seek strong and definite smells and tastes.

> **Example of gustatory sensory seeking behaviour that became a problem for a child with DME/2e:**
>
> One child who received occupational therapy for his sensory processing differences was surprised and relieved to find out that his love of and need to eat five to seven apples a day in addition to his normal meals could be labelled as taste sensory seeking behaviour. Whilst eating apples in general is very healthy, this child often got intense stomach cramps, but he did not think he could stop eating apples.
>
> With therapy, the child could identify that eating apples was an oral/mouth based sensory strategy he was using in overdrive to help him feel alert and "just right". This enabled him to explore other healthy foods as a strategy to help him feel regulated, but he also identified non-food related sensory strategies. With time he was able to eat a healthier amount of apples – pardon the irony!

The term **psychomotor overexcitabilities**[16] means having high levels of energy and being constantly on the go. The term describes children with DME/2e as almost always seeking more movement experiences than their peers. Through the lens of sensory processing differences, this will be described as sensory seeking behaviour with regards to the internal

Bridging the gap between sensory processing differences and overexcitabilities

Sensory differences	HLP overexcitabilities
Sensory over responsive (avoider)	Sensual: • **Sound** • **Visual images** • **Touch** • Smell & Taste (less)
Sensory seeking (craver)	Sensual: • **Smell** • **Taste** • Sound, Visual images, Touch (less) Psychomotor: • **Movement** • **Heavy work**

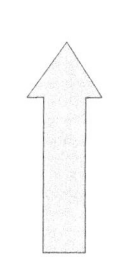

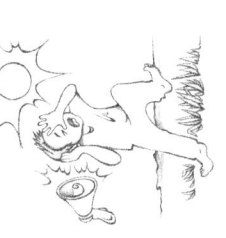

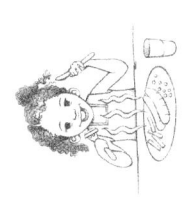

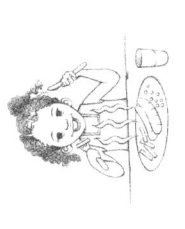

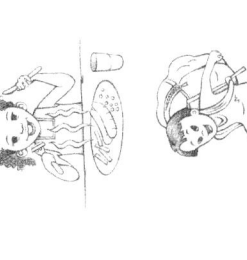

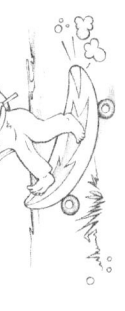

Figure 5.4 Bridging the gap between sensory processing differences and overexcitabilities, M. Ferreira, R. Howell.

Copyright material from Mariza Ferreira and Rebecca Howell (2024), *Occupational Therapy for Children with DME or Twice Exceptionality*, Routledge

vestibular and proprioceptive sensory systems. However, it is important to be aware that children with high learning potential may display increased sensory seeking behaviour with regards to movement and touch when they are intellectually bored, or when they feel agitated and/or when they are excited about something – but to a lesser extent in case of the latter two examples.

To understand these correlations better in a visual format, please refer to Figure 5.4, "Bridging the gap between sensory processing differences and overexcitabilities", which was developed as part of the DME-C therapy approach.

Sensory Based Motor Disorders

Sensory based motor disorders are divided into the subtypes postural disorder and dyspraxia, meaning the child has sensory-motor challenges. A child can have either postural disorder or dyspraxia (motor planning problems), and they often occur together.

Postural disorder

Postural disorder can be described as poor postural control and is when a child has difficulty getting into and maintaining a stable body position to engage in motor actions such as sitting at a desk to write or walking and running. Generally, children with postural disorder do not have a strong or stable body core and have poor body awareness. These children will often slouch or sprawl in their seats, hook their feet around chair legs and/or lean against walls when standing. They appear clumsy and often drop items, fall over their own feet, tire easily and also give up easily with motor tasks.

Dyspraxia

Dyspraxia is the difficulty to perform motor tasks in a smooth and coordinated way, especially new motor tasks. The child has difficulty with one or a combination of the steps of praxis or motor planning. These steps are:

- Ideation, which is the ability to grasp the idea of a new movement and to allow purposeful interaction with the environment, in other words "knowing what to do with an object and being able to anticipate a plan of action"
- Motor programming, which is the ability to plan and structure movements involving the motor and sensory systems. It involves knowing how to move and being able to send the right messages from the brain to relevant muscles and areas of the sensory system to carry out the movements
- Performance (or execution), which is carrying out the movement and putting the plan into action

A child with dyspraxia may appear clumsy and drop objects, bump into others, master age-related skills later than their peers and, once mastered, perform these skills with varying success from day to day, for example with handwriting. Children with dyspraxia often struggle to generalise skills. For example, they may be able to do their school shoelaces at home but struggle to do it when dressing after a physical education lesson; and they often have reduced confidence in new situations.

As discussed in Chapter 4, we view dyspraxia as part of developmental coordination disorder (see developmental coordination disorder or DCD, including dyspraxia).

Sensory Discrimination Disorder

Sensory discrimination disorder is when a child has difficulty distinguishing one sensation from another or knowing what a sensation means. This will make them appear awkward when participating in motor tasks in learning environments or in social situations.

Examples of difficulties with sensory discrimination are:

- When handling objects, a child may not know how much force to use, such as pressing too hard when writing - causing early hand muscle fatigue - or not pressing down hard enough (proprioception)
- When interacting with others, a child may not be able to tell when their body/skin has come into contact with another, resulting in the child appearing unaware of others' personal space (tactile)
- When communicating with others, a child may miss facial expressions and gestures or have difficulty in understanding what they mean, resulting in possible misunderstandings. They may also struggle to identify letters correctly, impacting on reading and learning (visual)
- When listening to others, a child may have difficulty distinguishing between sounds at the end of words, causing confusion when having to follow instructions (auditory)
- When eating, the child may be unable to tell how much food is in their mouth or when to swallow, indicating a possible choking hazard (tactile and gustatory)

Best Therapy Approach to Help Children with HLP who have Sensory Processing Differences

Important

Sensory processing differences, whilst described in literature in linear format to aid understanding (as in Miller's Sensory Processing Disorder Model, Dunn's Model of Sensory Processing, etc.), are by no means as simple in real life. Some children may have straightforward presentations of difficulties, whilst others have a complex combination of needs.

When the main areas of concern for a child with DME/2e and sensory processing differences relate to sensory modulation or sensory processing patterns, then we recommend the DME-C therapy approach is implemented.

When the main areas of concern relate to **sensory based motor disorders** (postural disorder and/or dyspraxia/DCD) and/or **sensory discrimination disorder**, we recommend therapists continue using the therapy approach or approaches they are familiar with, ensuring it is underpinned by a strong cognitive element and accompanied by the 10 Golden Nuggets we will discuss in Chapter 6, to improve the chances of successful therapy outcomes when working with children with DME/2e. Also, much of what we have recommended in the sections "Best therapy approach to help children with HLP and difficulties related to DCD", "Best therapy approach to help children with HLP who are also autistic" and "Best therapy approach to help children with HLP who also have ADHD" in Chapter 4, will be of relevance here too.

Conclusion

Now that therapists have read Chapters 4 and 5, we hope they will understand we are not against using any particular therapy approach to help children with DME/2e, as long as therapy meets the goals set at the start of the process, has a cognitive element, considers the 10 Golden Nuggets (see Chapter 6) and the 4 Essential Components (see Chapter 7). Therapy should also allow for active decision making from the child with the support of their family or carers, as well as involvement from their wider support network.

References

1. Ayres, A. J. (1977a). *Cluster analyses of measures of sensory integration.* The American Journal of Occupational Therapy, 31(6), 362-366.
Ayres, A. J., & Mailloux, Z. (1981). *Influence of sensory integration procedures on language development.* The American Journal of Occupational Therapy: Official Publication of the American Occupational Therapy Association, 35(6), 383-390. https://doi.org/10.5014/ajot.35.6.383.
2. Ayres, A. J. (1972). *Sensory integration and learning disorders.* WPS.
3. Miller J. L., Nielson M. D., Schoen A. S. (2012). *Attention deficit hyperactivity disorder and sensory modulation disorder: a comparison of behavior and physiology.* Res. Dev. Disabil. 33, 804-818 10.1016/j.ridd.2011.12.005.
4. Dunn, W. (1997) *The Impact of Sensory Processing Abilities on the Daily Lives of Young Children and Their Families: A Conceptual Model.* Infants & Young Children: April 1997, Volume 9, Issue 4, 23-35.
Royal College of Occupational Therapists Informed (2021) *Sensory Integration and sensory-based interventions* [Evidence Impact Spotlight].
5. Galiana-Simal, A., Muñoz-Martinez, V., & Beato-Fernandez, L. (2017). *Connecting eating disorders and sensory processing disorder: A sensory eating disorder hypothesis.* Global Journal of Intellectual and Developmental Disabilities, 3(4), 1-3.
6. Egger, H. L., & Emde, R. N. (2011). *Developmentally-sensitive diagnostic criteria for mental health disorders in early childhood: DSM-IV, RDC-PA, and the revised DC: 0-3.* American Psychologist, 66(2), 95-106.
7. Greenspan, S. I., & Wieder, S. (2008). *The interdisciplinary council on developmental and learning disorders diagnostic manual for infants and young children – An overview.* Journal of the Canadian Academy of Child and Adolescent Psychiatry, 17(2), 76-89.

8 Chien, C. W., Rodger, S., Copley, J., Branjerdporn, G., & Taggart, C. (2016). *Sensory processing and its relationship with children's daily life participation.* Physical & Occupational Therapy In Pediatrics, 36(1), 73–87.
Corbett, B. A., Muscatello, R. A., & Blain, S. D. (2016). *Impact of sensory sensitivity on physiological stress response and novel peer interaction in children with and without autism spectrum disorder.* Frontiers in Neuroscience, 10, 278.
Crozier, S. C., Goodson, J. Z., Mackay, M. L., Synnes, A. R., Grunau, R. E., Miller, S. P., & Zwicker, J. G. (2016). *Sensory processing patterns in children born very preterm.* The American Journal of Occupational Therapy, 70(1), 1–7.
9 Miller J. L., Nielson M. D., Schoen A. S. (2012). Attention deficit hyperactivity disorder and sensory modulation disorder: a comparison of behavior and physiology. *Res. Dev. Disabil.* 33, 804–818 10.1016/j.ridd.2011.12.005.
OR Bialer D., Miller. L.J. (2012). *No Longer A Secret: Unique Common Sense Strategies for Children with Sensory or Motor Challenges.* Future Horizons.
10 Dunn, W. (1997) *The Impact of Sensory Processing Abilities on the Daily Lives of Young Children and Their Families: A Conceptual Model.* Infants & Young Children: April 1997, Volume 9, Issue 4, 23–35.
11 Jarrard, P. (2008) *Sensory Issues in Gifted Children: Synthesis of the Literature.* Retrieved from: https://sensoryhealth.org/sites/default/files/publications/SensoryissuesinGiftedChildren.pdf.
12 Piechowski, M. M., & Miller, N. B. (1995). Assessing developmental potential in gifted children: A comparison of methods. Roeper Review: A Journal on Gifted Education, 17(3), 176–180. https://doi.org/10.1080/02783199509553654.
13 Jarrard, P. (2022). *Sensory Issues in Gifted Children: Synthesis of the Literature.* Retrieved from https://www.spdstar.org/sites/default/files/publications/SensoryissuesinGiftedChildren.pdf.
14 Bainbridge, C. (2020, June 11) *Dabrowski's overexcitabilities in gifted children.* Retrieved on July 9, 2022 from www.verywellfamily.com/dabrowskis-overexcitabilities-in-gifted-children-1449118.
Alias A, Rahman S, Majid RA, Yassin SFM. *Dabrowski's Overexcitabilities Profile among Gifted Students.* Asian Social Science. 2013;9(16). doi:10.5539/ass.v9n16p120.
15 Bainbridge, C. (2020, June 11) *Dabrowski's overexcitabilities in gifted children.* Retrieved on July 9, 2022 from www.verywellfamily.com/dabrowskis-overexcitabilities-in-gifted-children-1449118.
Alias A, Rahman S, Majid RA, Yassin SFM. *Dabrowski's Overexcitabilities Profile among Gifted Students.* Asian Social Science. 2013;9(16). doi:10.5539/ass.v9n16p120.
16 Bainbridge, C. (2020, June 11) *Dabrowski's overexcitabilities in gifted children.* Retrieved on July 9, 2022 from www.verywellfamily.com/dabrowskis-overexcitabilities-in-gifted-children-1449118.
Alias A, Rahman S, Majid RA, Yassin SFM. *Dabrowski's Overexcitabilities Profile among Gifted Students.* Asian Social Science. 2013;9(16). doi:10.5539/ass.v9n16p120.

Chapter six
The DME-C Approach's Foundation
The 10 Golden Nuggets

Introduction

This chapter begins by exploring and answering some of the common concerns of occupational therapists new to the world of working with children with DME/2e. Following this, we introduce the DME-C therapy approach by discussing the foundation it is built on: the 10 Golden Nuggets. These are the principles by which occupational therapists can start to tailor their support for children with DME/2e.

Questions or Concerns OTs May Have

The concerns or questions Mariza had as an occupational therapist at the time she started to work with children with DME/2e are probably similar to the ones readers currently have. To name a few, these may be along the lines of:

- I have never heard of DME or 2e before. How can I possibly help and advise on the issues that children with DME/2e face?
- The people in my professional network, including my colleagues, have never heard about DME/2e or do not believe it exists. How will I approach the subject with them and get them onboard?
- How do I spot a child with DME/2e?
- DME/2e is not a recognised condition. How can I comfortably refer to this in reports?
- I am having limited success with therapy. Where can I find more information and guidance on helping children with DME/2e?
- The children with DME/2e I work with can be very challenging. How do I deal with this?
- The parents of the children with DME/2e I work with are very involved with regards to their child's therapy and education. How do I deal with this?
- The terminology that parents of children with DME/2e use to describe their challenges can be very confusing. How can I make sense of it?
- I am gaining confidence in myself and the knowledge that I can help children with DME/2e. But what happens when the help they need is outside of my remit or scope? Where do I refer them on to?
- Occupational therapists are well suited to help children with DME/2e. But why is our role generally unrecognised?

The good news is that all of these questions are answered in this book to help readers become familiar with HLP, DME/2e, the DME-C therapy approach and the other advice and

DOI: 10.4324/9781003334033-6

guidance we give. Some of these questions are answered in other parts of the book, but we will summarise here our thoughts about those not directly addressed elsewhere.

DME/2e is not a recognised condition

We are mindful of the fact that DME/2e in itself is not a recognised condition in the *Diagnostic and Statistical Manual of Mental Disorders, Fifth Edition* (DSM-V) or the *International Statistical Classification of Diseases and Related Health Problems* (ICD-11). However, the same can be said for sensory processing disorder (SPD), and this does not deter occupational therapists and other professionals from acknowledging its existence or the fact that people with SPD need help to deal with related participation challenges.

Similarly, whilst DME/2e is not formally recognised, it certainly exists; children with DME/2e have unique difficulties and participation challenges in the activities that are important to them. We recommend occupational therapists view and use DME/2e as a term to describe and better understand a child's profile. Whilst it forms part of neurodiversity, it is important to still refer to DME/2e by name to increase awareness of this part of a child's profile. Not doing so runs the risk of either or both important aspects of a child's profile being ignored and overlooked, meaning that accommodations for the child's high cognitive abilities and/or support for their SEND or learning difficulty may not be made.

Colleagues and other professionals have not heard of DME/2e or do not believe it exists

We are aware that, despite widespread evidence that DME/2e exists,[1] some people have a hard time accepting it and may continue to deny it. In her book *Parenting Dual Exceptional Children* author Denise Yates says,[2]

> let us assume for a moment that they are right, that there is no such thing as DME. Treating children and young people as if they *did* have DME and supporting them in a strengths-based approach may still be no bad thing, especially if it motivated them to be their best version of themselves.

Indeed, a strength-based approach is known to work well for children with DME/2e.[3] Working with someone who does not believe DME/2e exists can be difficult, but it is not a lost cause. It will, however, take some effort to find a way forward and work collaboratively. Yates gives good tips and hints for parents of children with DME/2e on how to engage with their child's school in the book chapter "Positive relationships with the professionals" and this, as well as the whole book, is an informative guide to the children in question.

For occupational therapists, it helps to have as much evidence as possible regarding a child's profile: their characteristics, their strengths and their challenges. Occupational therapists are able to identify much of the latter two through assessment and the former from working with the child. However, it is also extremely valuable to get information regarding a child's cognitive ability from other professional reports such as those done by educational psychologists and/or organisations such as Mensa or Potential Plus UK. The facts and advice contained in these reports support occupational therapists' and others' understanding of the child's profile, and we can then highlight the term DME/2e to describe the profile (high learning potential together with a SEND). Occupational therapists can support the parents or carers of a child with DME/2e to advocate for their child by guiding them on how to explain their child's profile to others. Occupational therapists can also support parents and carers by attending meetings, etc. with them. We would recommend that supporting parents to advocate through guiding them to explain their child's profile empowers parents better, whereas attending meetings with them may create an over-dependence on therapists. Remember that whoever is advocating for the child needs to always keep the child's needs at the forefront of any communication with a "doubter", emphasising these needs above a diagnosis or belief in a particular profile. This way we will guard against getting into a battle of beliefs and make sure people are on the same page of supporting the child's needs. This is much more likely to win the person over, ultimately benefiting the child.

The role of occupational therapists to help children with DME/2e is generally unrecognised

We are of the opinion that occupational therapy for children with DME/2e is **vital** to helping them with whatever occupational performance challenges they face. However, occupational therapy is often part of a wider solution that involves other professionals and agencies. We therefore strongly believe in multidisciplinary teamworking where this would clearly be beneficial and is possible.

As with any new SEND, condition or profile that occupational therapists come across in their work with children, they can supplement their existing knowledge and further their training in that particular area, whether by formal or informal means, in order to have a positive impact on children's lives. Working holistically with children is ingrained in the approach of a paediatric occupational therapist, and this allows us to see how a child's strengths and challenges affect every area of their lives, working with them towards independence in the specific occupational performance areas important to them. This makes us, or should make us, leading professionals when working with children with DME/2e. Yet, most people in the gifted/DME/2e communities are unaware of the many benefits occupational therapy can bring for children with DME/2e.

It could be the case that one of the main reasons for the role of occupational therapy being unrecognised is that many therapists are dogged by imposter syndrome. Our observations are that, certainly in the UK, many qualified and/or experienced occupational therapists seem to suffer from imposter syndrome, which prevents them from speaking up. This curtails occupational therapy being understood and acknowledged by other professionals for the myriad and powerful benefits it can offer. We suspect this may be the case in other occupational therapy communities and cultures as well. Imposter syndrome[4] is when a person believes that they are not as competent as others perceive them to be. An individual with imposter syndrome feels like a fraud and that they may be "found out" at any moment.

People experience imposter syndrome regardless of their degree, expertise, work background or skill level. Occupational therapists who have imposter syndrome may not feel confident to help children with DME/2e despite having or gaining the "tools" to do so, and when they do work with these children, they may not feel confident enough to support them beyond the immediate therapy setting. We are of the opinion that the more therapists face and address their own imposter syndrome, the more they will feel empowered to speak up for their clients and speak out about the essential role of occupational therapy.

There are various ways for a person to address their imposter syndrome, and everyone's journey will be different. There is a lot of helpful information widely available on the topic, and we advocate the general advice to learn more about what imposter syndrome is, recognise the signs in oneself, understand that it is quite common among professionals and actively address it. Some successful strategies to achieve this are to talk about imposter syndrome with a mentor, track one's own professional development regarding further knowledge and skills in the area of DME/2e, purposefully use positive self-talk when negative self-talk about our abilities as therapists are prevalent and embrace imposter syndrome as a motivator to take on the new opportunities of helping children with DME/2e.[5]

Having been to many international conferences in the UK and Europe attended by professionals who work with children with high learning potential and DME/2e, we have not come across any other occupational therapists and believe that none had attended previously. Colleagues initially viewed us with scepticism, but when they learned how we can and have helped children with DME/2e, their attitudes changed to ones of appreciation and hope, as well as wishing they had known about the benefits of occupational therapy long before. They often expressed the desire to know more about what it could bring to the conversation.

As occupational therapists grow in their knowledge and experience, so will their ability to advocate for the needs of children with DME/2e. It is our experience that with developing confidence, opportunities to explain the importance of occupational therapy for this group of children arise and, in turn, more families with children with DME/2e seek out support.

The 10 Golden Nuggets

The raw materials that make up the **foundation** of the DME-C therapy approach are called the 10 Golden Nuggets and are concerned with the **method** in which occupational therapists provide therapy. The 10 Golden Nuggets relate to the non-OT factors we discussed in Chapter 4, and although they were "discovered" when working with children with DME/2e who have challenges relating to sensory processing, unhelpful thought patterns and self-regulation, many are also relevant when working with children with DME/2e who have other SENDs and occupational performance challenges. The 10 Golden Nuggets are essential to fostering a strengths-based and effective therapy approach. Their importance cannot be emphasised enough. Please refer to Figure 6.1, The DME-C therapy approach's foundation: The 10 Golden Nuggets, which provides a summary that can be printed off for easy reference. We will explain each Golden Nugget further, which will provide more clarity about why each one is important.

The DME-C therapy approach's foundation: The 10 Golden Nuggets	
Golden Nugget 1. Purposefully empower parents/carers alongside children	**Golden Nugget** 2. Lengthen the sessions
Golden Nugget 3. Set clear & healthy boundaries from the start	**Golden Nugget** 4. Use direct language
Golden Nugget 5. Monitor your responses	**Golden Nugget** 6. Do not repeat previously learned information
Golden Nugget 7. To make sessions engaging: Include practical and cipher activities	**Golden Nugget** 8. To make sessions engaging: Design unexpected or delayed outcomes
Golden Nugget 9. Find the WOW and Super WOW Factors	**Golden Nugget** 10. Foster a growth mindset

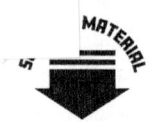

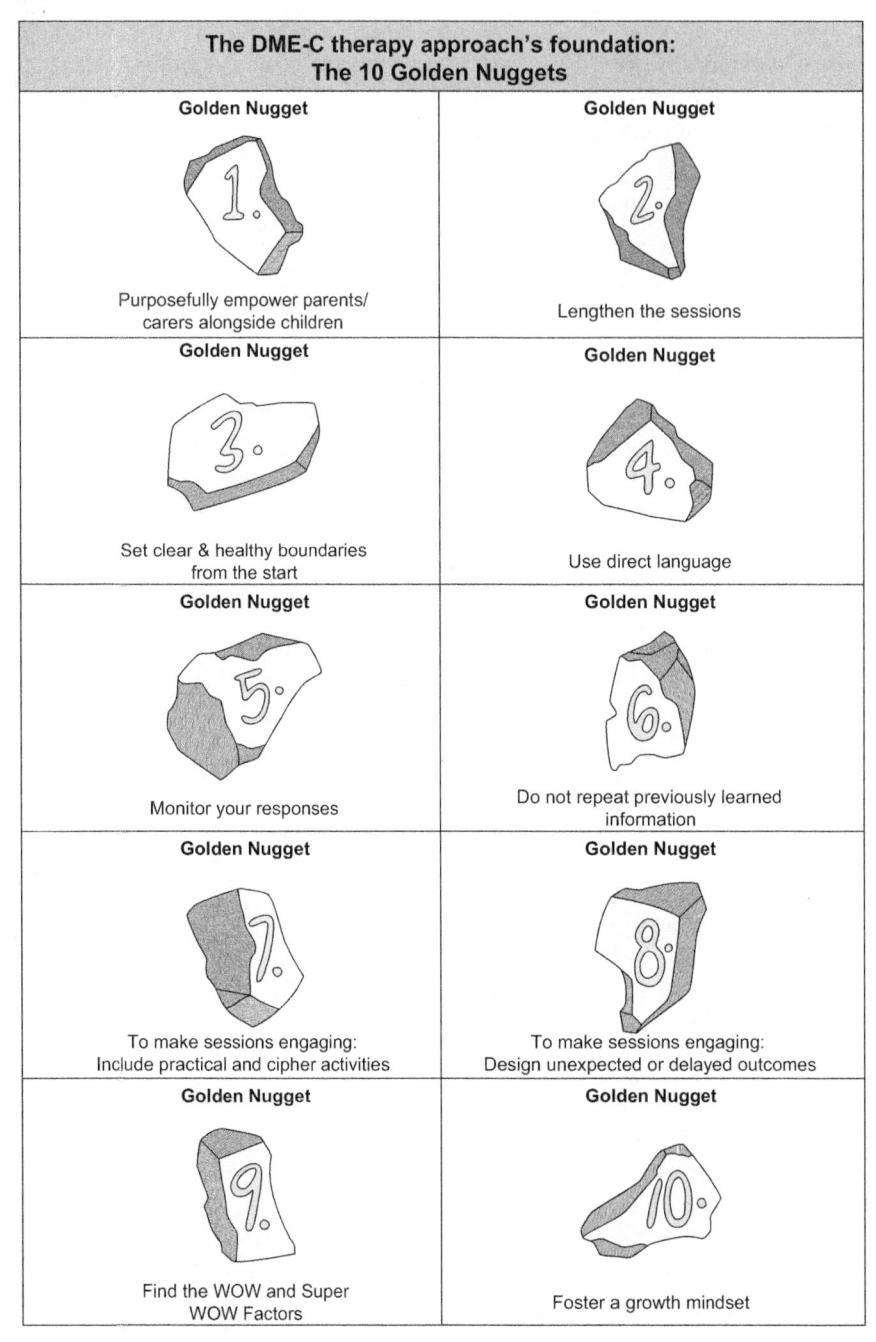

Figure 6.1 The DME-C therapy approach's foundation: The 10 Golden Nuggets, M. Ferreira, R. Howell.

Copyright material from Mariza Ferreira and Rebecca Howell (2024), *Occupational Therapy for Children with DME or Twice Exceptionality*, Routledge

Golden Nugget 1: Purposefully empower parents/carers alongside children

Occupational therapists should be realistic about the fact that they only work with children with DME/2e for a number of sessions over what is essentially a short period of time. It is therefore important they find ways to ensure their input has maximum impact, that the skills and strategies they are helping children with can be transferred to the children's everyday lives and that it can be understood by those supporting them such as their parents and teachers.

At its nature, occupational therapy is client-centred, and children are by default empowered through the occupational therapy process when it is directed at addressing areas of occupational performance which are important to them. Furthermore, by providing therapy on a one-to-one basis, children can be confident therapists have the capacity to help them address areas of difficulties that are highly individual to them. As mentioned in Chapter 1, the introduction of the book, conducting sessions on a one-to-one basis also enables therapists to maintain a high level of observation and awareness of children during sessions which allows them to guide sessions appropriately.

Occupational therapists further empower children and their parents or carers by making sure they understand everyone is on the same team. Whilst occupational therapists are the ones with the knowledge and skills to help children with DME/2e, they need to view the children and their parents/carers as partners in the therapy process – acknowledging that they know best about what would work or not work for them. They may also already have ideas and strategies they find helpful, so exploring what all parties have to bring, and how this can be combined, will not only add vital information to the process but will also mean children and parents/carers feel valued and are more likely to accept what therapists are suggesting.

A practical way to ensure therapists are empowering a child's parents or carers is to allow them to be part of sessions as observers and as contributors when invited to participate as the therapist deems appropriate. Their role needs to be communicated to parents separately prior to therapy starting. Not communicating this may mean parents get involved to the extent of taking over in sessions.

In most cases it is appropriate for parents or carers to participate in therapy sessions, but there may be occasions when therapists identify, either before therapy commences or as it progresses, that it is not in the child's best interest for parents and carers to continue participating. In our experience, when the therapist briefly explains the reasons, parents are receptive to this change in plan, as they understand it is needed for their child to gain maximum benefit from sessions.

An example of when it may not be appropriate for a parent or carer to participate in sessions is when the child and parent have a strained relationship which has progressed to the point of both parties having heightened emotions, clouding sessions. Whilst some misunderstandings between a parent and child can be used effectively in therapy to illustrate how interactions with others have an impact on emotional regulation, where these are more serious, therapists will need to evaluate whether addressing such misunderstandings falls within their remit or scope and whether it would be better addressed by a psychologist, family therapist or other similarly trained professional.

If parents or carers are not participating in sessions for the reason mentioned above or perhaps if participation is not possible due to work or other childcare commitments, then it is still important for therapists to keep them informed of issues addressed during sessions. Therapists have different ways of doing this, with verbal and/or written feedback being some of the most common ones. We have found that keeping parents and carers informed and involved throughout the therapy process, and addressing any questions they have along the way, has the best chance of successful therapy outcomes.

Another way to empower parents or carers is to encourage them to develop a deeper understanding of sensory processing differences, how it relates to their child with DME/2e and how they can help them further. Doing courses on the topic in-person or online, such as the ones on https://www.theotcompany.com/online-courses/, are some popular options. Parents tend to either do them prior to therapy starting or alongside the therapy process.

Golden Nugget 2: Lengthen the sessions

As explained in Chapter 2, in general children with HLP or giftedness have a large capacity to take in information, make connections between concepts and have a desire to understand those concepts on a deeper level. This means they can usually concentrate for longer periods of time than their peers, with the exception of perhaps children with DME/2e who have ADHD and who struggle with sustained focus in certain situations. This thirst for knowledge or "intellectual overexcitability" usually announces itself very early on in the therapy process and has both positive and negative sides. When managed correctly by the therapist, these characteristics can all be used to support the child to gain the most from therapy.

The positive side of a child with DME/2e's intellectual overexcitability and associated ability to concentrate for longer is that in most cases they can cope with the introduction of more than one idea or concept at a time and at a faster pace than their peers. They also have the capacity to participate in longer therapy sessions. Indeed, once on-task children with DME/2e do better with longer sessions than with breaking the activity sooner, which often results in frustration as they often feel like they have just started delving deeper into the concepts. We have found the benefits of longer sessions holds true even for children with DME/2e as young as five or six years of age. We would therefore recommend that, if therapists are able to and have the capacity within themselves, they conduct double therapy sessions. As a guideline, a double session lasts about one and a half hours each, whereas single sessions are considered to be 45 minutes each.

The negative side of a child with DME/2e's insatiable thirst for knowledge is that, while they relish learning new things, it is often hard for them to implement the techniques and strategies they have learnt in sessions into their everyday lives. In fact, it may take several therapy sessions before they begin to really see the benefit of implementing what they have learnt. We believe one of the reasons is because children with DME/2e enjoy the cognitive element of learning new concepts (a strength) more than actually implementing the strategies, as this means facing their particular challenges. Another reason may relate to their perfectionist traits and fear of failure – such as being afraid of not choosing the "best" activities to address their sensory processing differences and therefore not choosing any. So, even if they request one full day of therapy to cover the whole program (yes, it has happened!), it is important to explain that time is needed between sessions both for reflection and implementation.

We would therefore recommend that therapy sessions themselves are spaced out ideally two weeks apart. Longer than this may mean you lose some momentum with therapy. However, this is sometimes inevitable due to therapist and/or child availability, which can be impacted by factors such as holidays, sickness or other unforeseen circumstances. Therapists can build momentum again, but this may mean compromising on Golden Nugget 6. However, if done creatively, such as by asking the child to share their thoughts on the concepts that were covered in previous sessions and filling in the gaps, therapists will still have the child's willingness to participate fully in sessions. Therapists can also consider spacing sessions one week apart, but in cases like this the child needs to have a high level of motivation to not just participate fully in sessions but also to complete the tasks set between sessions at home.

In the case of a child with DME/2e who has ADHD, following their initial full assessment of the child, therapists need to consider whether the child will be able to cope with single or double sessions. The former is likely to be appropriate, with the latter being considered when the child can hyperfocus in sessions and has the ability to transition out of sessions in a timely manner.

To summarise, ideally, have double sessions (of one and a half hours each) two weeks apart. But remember that this decision should be guided by the particular child with DME/2e's individual needs.

Golden Nugget 3: Set clear and healthy boundaries from the start

A boundary is defined[6] as "a real or imagined line that marks the edge or limit of something" or "the limit of what someone considers to be acceptable behaviour". The concept of setting boundaries with children has been around for a very long time, and has been discussed, studied and debated a million times over in literature, in the media, among parents and anyone who has ever had some kind of responsibility towards a child, whether that be a teacher, therapist, coach, club manager, nanny or childminder etc. People view setting boundaries very individually with opinions ranging from no or few boundaries being needed, to strict and rigid boundaries and everything in between. Children with SEND often struggle to meet expectations set by adults, and this means boundaries may be tested more often by these children than those who are neurotypical. There is much to debate in this arena, however, we want to guide here as we feel it is appropriate to take into account the needs of children with DME/2e.

We appreciate that every therapist has a unique personality and believe the authenticity they bring to the therapeutic relationship with a child as a result of this in itself contributes to successful therapy outcomes. In addition to this, we have found that having considered and appropriate healthy boundaries from the start of the therapy process is very important, as they create a sense of safety and trust.[7] They also help towards the development of a sense of self for the child,[8] self-control and learning how to build good relationships with others.

Having healthy boundaries in the therapist/child relationship is always important, but it is especially true when working with children with DME/2e since there are some additional challenges around them. They may not make the same assumptions about boundaries as neurotypical children and so could fall foul of a boundary without intending to. Due to their creativity, emotional intensity and advanced language skills, children with DME/2e can often argue convincingly about the need for boundaries.[9] However, children with DME/2e are much more likely to respect the boundaries if they understand the reasons for them, which in turn helps them to have more insight into the impact of their actions and where they need to draw the line in otherwise ambiguous situations.

Bearing these factors in mind, therapists working with children with DME/2e should ensure that boundaries are thought through in advance as much as possible, have no logical holes, and that they themselves understand the reasons for them and can articulate them. Boundaries may look different from one therapist to another but, together with their reasons, should be clearly stated in a non-threatening way from the start of the interaction with a child. Boundaries should then be stuck to as far as possible, although a reason or need for renegotiation may become apparent over time. When this happens, therapists should not keep blindly stating the boundary but genuinely listen to the child's concerns, state their own and come up with a solution together that meets the concerns of both parties, if possible. Most importantly, boundaries should always be set with the understanding that the therapist is on the child's team, wants to work with them and help them to develop their skills.

Setting healthy boundaries is a two-way street. It effectively means telling the child what type of behaviour the therapist is comfortable with in sessions and what they are not, and the child also telling the therapist what they are comfortable with and what they are not. Respecting each other's boundaries has the positive consequence that both therapist and child are able to work towards the goal of helping the child develop effective strategies for the issues they want to address in therapy. Not respecting the boundaries has the negative consequence that the therapist and child may not be able to work towards those goals. It is important for the child to know this, and that the choice is theirs.

Any child an occupational therapist works with will use creative ways to determine how far they can "push the boundaries". Children do this because they want to know if they can trust the therapist. And if they can, they can feel safe with the therapist. And if they feel safe, they can work on the therapy goals they have set. However, it has been our experience that a child with DME/2e may push the boundaries harder or for longer, particularly if they have already developed a general distrust of authority figures in their lives, as we discussed in Chapter 4. Therapists need to be mindful of this and should consider that oppositional and/or confrontational behaviour, whether in the form of the "instant explosion" or "slow burner", is not necessarily an attempt to get out of therapy, especially if children are truly motivated to work on the goals they have set. In fact, it may be their "test" to see if the therapist will stick with the boundaries set, and whether it is worth their time to work with her. In other words, they need a therapist to "put their actions where their mouth is".

Some boundaries that we have found helpful in therapy sessions relate to how the therapist and the child communicate with each other, how the therapist and child communicate with a parent or carer who is observing sessions and what is expected in terms of the child's interaction with the therapy space and therapy equipment.

Therapists may therefore communicate that they expect everyone in a session, including children and parents, to speak kindly to each other, without swearing, and that differing opinions are welcomed but should be communicated respectfully. The therapist should also invite the child to share whether there is anything in particular they like or dislike with regards to communication – such as not being called a diminutive form of their name or not being touched physically – as in the case of sensory tactile defensiveness. Therapists should be mindful that children may not yet know how to convey their communication preferences effectively and that this is likely to improve over the course of therapy as they learn how to advocate for themselves.

With regards to the therapy space and equipment, therapists may want to communicate that this is to be treated with care, so it can be used by other children and by them in future sessions. This is because children with DME/2e, like all children, may sometimes choose to use destructive behaviour to convey feelings of frustration when their words fail them. It is therefore prudent to explain to the child that the therapist knows things are sometimes so frustrating that it may feel they want to break something; but when this happens, they need to tell the therapist or give some prearranged sign, so they can get some time out (or whatever is agreed beforehand will help the child).

When therapists encounter situations during sessions that relate to pre-set boundaries, it is easier to enforce those boundaries and deal with the issue which has led to the boundary being pushed in the first place, as opposed to when no boundaries have been set. For example, a child who deliberately starts to break therapy equipment can be reminded of the agreement to tell the therapist they are frustrated, and the real reason for that frustration can be explored. However, there are times when a boundary has to be created on the spot, such as when a child deliberately tries to disrupt a session.

An example of a therapist creating an instant boundary

A therapist worked with a twelve-year-old child who could be described as an "instant explosion" from the start of therapy. The child had a history of confrontational behaviour with adults, but the therapist believed this to partly stem from feeling constantly misunderstood by others and insecurity, with subsequent controlling behaviour in any

> situations that seemed threatening. The child had previously said they wanted to work with the therapist to improve their ability to self-regulate.
>
> At the start of one of the sessions, the therapist asked the child to do a craft activity with her, stating that she would help the child with any of the "fiddly bits" of the activity (the child also had some poor fine motor skills).
>
> Initially the child seemed keen to complete the activity, but then picked up the table and chair and moved it to the edge of the therapy room, stating they did not want to do the activity. The therapist realised an instant boundary had to be created, so explained to the child that the activity was chosen to help the child develop their self-regulation skills and gave a choice about how they could participate; they could choose to do it either at the edge of the room, or carry the table and chair back to its original place and do the activity there.
>
> The child continued to argue, saying, "No, there is a third option. I just will not do it" and being generally unkind and challenging in their behaviour. The therapist spoke calmly to reinforce the boundary and explained they understood some of the feelings they were having about the task, being specific about these, saying, "I think you don't want to do this because you will find it hard to do and that is why you are behaving like this". She also reassured the child she was not going to give up on the child despite their oppositional and challenging behaviour. It needed several rounds of a similar exchange until the child agreed to complete the activity, saying, "Fine, but I'll do it here". The child proceeded to enjoy the activity. The therapist reported that although it was a difficult situation, this was the first major breakthrough in building trust with the child.

Always remember the therapist is the one responsible for therapy sessions and the direction it needs to go in to achieve the goals that have been set at the start of therapy. Children with DME/2e can be particularly good at subtly steering situations away from facing tough issues (even though they want to work on them!). Therapists need to be mindful of this and resist the urge to be swept away with wherever the child is taking them, unless they believe it will be conducive to the therapy process and helping the child.

Golden Nuggets 4 and 5: Use direct language and Monitor your responses

In our experience, children with DME/2e are generally much more direct in their communication style than other children. This can result in them easily offending others, as if they have a lack of consideration for others' feelings or awareness of social nuances. While the latter may be true in certain cases, such as children with HLP who are autistic and who struggle to read social situations, most children with DME/2e just want to get straight to the point because of their intellectual and emotional overexcitabilities.

There are some cultures where a very direct style of communication is welcomed and where therapists can use it effectively from the outset of the therapy process, but this is not the case in the English culture and perhaps the rest of the UK. In fact, we believe this is often the reason why children with HLP and DME/2e are misunderstood by others, especially by adults who may view them as disrespectful, rude or odd.

As therapists, we may find ourselves surprised and even offended by how direct children with DME/2e communicate with us. But therapists need to remember the children mean no harm by it, should consciously choose not to take offence or let it alter their attitude towards the child, and can use it to their advantage in therapy sessions.

When therapists are aware of or watching their own "offence register" and monitoring their own personal responses to it, using a direct style of communication with a child with DME/2e can be one of the most effective tools in the therapeutic relationship. In practice this means therapists should consider children with DME/2e's advanced intellectual abilities and therefore speak to them like equals and not "as children". Therapists should explain ideas and concepts at the level the child requires, even if this is more detailed than for other children, and not try to hide anything. Children with DME/2e are more likely to comply with the therapy process if they understand why they have to do something.

Therapists can also calmly verbalise or call out when they see the child behaving in unhealthy or inappropriate ways – whether the reason for this is their particular sensory processing differences, thought patterns, one of the non-OT factors or another reason. Therapists can then help the child find more appropriate coping strategies and/or techniques.

An example of using direct language and monitoring your responses

The mother of a six-year-old girl with confirmed HLP/giftedness, requested occupational therapy for her as she reported that she often had "meltdowns", "tantrums" and emotional outbursts which made family life difficult, affected her learning at school and her ability to make friends. The family thought this was mainly due to sensory processing differences.

The occupational therapy assessment confirmed the child had an overall profile of sensory sensitivity towards noise and touch, but she also had motor coordination difficulties. The child also displayed some of the non-OT factors commonly associated with children with HLP such as perfectionism, a highly developed sense of right and wrong and asynchronous development (a marked disparity between her high cognitive abilities and social skills development). The therapist also suggested they consider an assessment for autism, which the family later pursued and which was confirmed. The therapist hypothesised the child's outbursts were a result of all these aforementioned difficulties and agreed with the child and her mother to focus therapy on developing better coping strategies for her sensory issues and to explore unhealthy thought patterns that were contributing to her outbursts.

> During one therapy session in particular, which was approximately halfway into the therapy program and after much work had been done to help the child identify when she was dysregulated, she became upset about something the therapist had said. What followed was an emotional outburst with intense screaming and unintelligible vocalisation which was unexpected from a six-year-old child who otherwise had an excellent vocabulary and who could generally communicate well.
>
> The therapist reported that her immediate reaction was to feel offended, but at the same time recognised the child was displaying asynchronous development and that the behaviour could be addressed directly. The therapist was able to dial down her offence register and in between the child's screaming, calmly pointed out to the child that her behaviour showed that she was dysregulated. The therapist also gently suggested that in this, or in similar situations in the future, she could consider using some of the coping strategies she had been learning about in therapy. The child seemed surprised at the therapist's handling of the situation and calmly asked if she could have a break and go to the bathroom.
>
> While the child was outside the therapy room, the therapist asked the mother how she felt about the direct handling of the situation. The mother responded by saying they have been struggling for years to manage the child's explosive reactions to situations and that getting help to manage it, such as learning how to speak with her directly about it, was one of the reasons why they had sought therapy.
>
> This particular incident seemed to be a turning point for the child in the therapy program. When therapy concluded, her mother reported that occupational therapy was "very practical and also helped my child to help herself. Signposting to autism was also really useful. She is extremely good at masking but the therapist treated her exactly right for an autistic child with extremely high intelligence".

We encourage all therapists who work with children with DME/2e to consider using direct language with them during therapy, even if it does not come naturally. Many therapists we have trained say that this is one of the things they think they will struggle with the most, as they are afraid of coming across as authoritative, judgemental, inconsiderate or as if they are speaking down to the child, which could be damaging to the therapeutic relationship with the child. However, it is our experience that direct communication can be very effective if the therapist has first monitored his or her personal response and made a conscious adjustment of it if necessary, and always approaches the child from the viewpoint of everyone being on "team child".

Golden Nugget 6: Do not repeat previously learned information

Children with DME/2e learn rapidly, have excellent memory, reason well, have strong curiosity and are keen observers. This is why they can easily feel intellectually bored if information is not presented at a level which allows them to think things through, make connections between concepts, go deeper by considering implications and alternatives and categorise information in a way that makes sense to them.

As we discussed in Chapter 4, children with DME/2e who feel intellectually bored can display unacceptable or challenging behaviour in certain situations. We have found this to be true for therapy settings as well. In fact, this non-OT factor is one of the main reasons why we recommend against approaching therapy from a traditional occupational therapy viewpoint where "repetition" or "overlearning" play a significant part in therapy sessions.

Therapists may find that children with DME/2e who are motivated to develop better coping strategies for their sensory processing differences may initially be very engaged as new concepts are introduced and discussed in sessions. However, if these concepts are repeated and/or presented at the same level of depth in follow up sessions, the same children may suddenly seem annoyed or angry. They may disengage by way of avoiding eye contact, turning away or moving to the other side of the therapy space, be verbally aggressive or become destructive towards whatever objects or therapy equipment they can get their hands on. When this happens, the therapist should first consider whether the child's disengagement or aggressive behaviour stems from intellectual boredom. Children with DME/2e may outrightly question why something they have already learnt is being repeated, or they may agree that this is what bothers them if therapists offer it as a reason for their disengagement or destructive behaviour. Remember, as we discussed in the previous section, that it is okay for therapists to name the behaviour they see (in other words being direct in their communication with the child) as long as they have checked and adjusted their own offence registers.

We would recommend that therapists, at the start of the therapy process, give the child and parent/carer a rough outline of the concepts that will be addressed in therapy and how this will progress. For instance, the therapist can say that for the first few sessions the focus will be on exploring the child's sensory challenges and finding bespoke strategies to help them deal with them; whereafter, they will explore and address any unhelpful thought processes which may be affecting the child's ability to participate in everyday activities.

The therapist can explain that they will move rapidly through concepts without much repetition unless the child expressly asks for the therapist to repeat or explain certain concepts. The therapist can also explain that he or she anticipates the child may feel they want to skip over some information entirely, but that they should try and work through them regardless as all the concepts are related and necessary to help the child develop depth in their understanding of their particular challenges and how to address them.

Furthermore, the therapist should explain to the child and their parents or carers that they are teaching them the **fundamental concepts** of identifying their own sensory needs and thought processes impacting on activity participation, as well as the **principles of effective coping strategies**. This way the child and their family will have the tools to adapt their strategies to be age appropriate as the child grows and develops, long after therapy has stopped.

We may point out that although it is important not to repeat concepts directly in sessions with children with DME/2e, we do feel it is necessary for the child and their family to have a reminder of the concepts addressed during sessions for them to keep track of the coping strategies they find helpful in sessions and those they discover between sessions as part of their "therapy homework". We therefore recommend that therapists provide them with a written summary of the key points covered in a session and worksheets which they can complete between sessions.

The written summaries should be addressed to the child, and although it is our aim that they will read it, they should by no means be forced to do so. The summaries are also especially helpful for parents to reflect on afterwards and/or to share with the child's other parent or carer where applicable. They empower parents to better understand and advocate for their child's needs at school and in the wider community.

The worksheets are helpful as they encourage the child to move from just understanding or thinking about the concepts to actually developing their own coping strategies, which they are sometimes reluctant to do, as we discussed earlier. As the therapy program progresses, the child will build up a bank of activities or coping strategies which they can start using in different situations.

The summaries and initial coping strategies the children have developed also act as a refresher further down the line after therapy has stopped and they feel they need to revisit some of the concepts. In addition, they act as a springboard from which to develop new and more age appropriate strategies as the child develops.

We have come across some rare cases in which children with DME/2e have engaged well in sessions but have not been able or willing to complete the worksheets between sessions throughout the whole therapy process. Some children reported they "have it in their heads" or that they will do the homework in their own time. We have respected their decision as we view them as equal partners in the therapy process. In these situations, we have also offered to write a bespoke home program for them which combines the summaries of concepts covered and the worksheets, but only if they really wanted it. The children's parents have reported that they had engaged with the home programs although only with certain sections. We conclude that the children have gravitated towards the parts of the programs they felt the most comfortable with and which they felt ready for. Any part that is completed will represent progress for the child.

In Chapter 7 we will discuss the four walls, or "the 4 Essential Components" of D, M, E and C which form part of the DME-C therapy approach, and we will also provide some examples of session summaries we have used successfully in therapy. Please note these should be used as guides only, as each therapist's summaries will look different depending on the type of activities they choose to use in their sessions.

Golden Nuggets 7 and 8: To make sessions engaging: Include practical and cipher activities and Design unexpected or delayed outcomes

Chinese Confucian philosopher Xun Kuang said, "Tell me and I forget. Teach me and I may remember. Involve me and I learn". We could not have said it better, and in the DME-C approach we therefore place a strong emphasis on using practical activities that have an element of mystery and/or novelty during sessions to explain concepts and illustrate points. Furthermore, we have found that this "messing with their heads" sometimes helps to lift the mood for children with DME/2e who take themselves and the world very seriously. However, this should be done with sensitivity on the part of the therapist; not all children with DME/2e respond well to this approach due to their personality type. It is difficult to tell how they will respond in advance, so we recommend trying it with all and being sensitive to the response.

Due to the rapid progression of the therapy process with a child with DME/2e where therapists address the child's sensory processing differences, unhelpful thought patterns and self-regulation impacting on their activity participation, the general rule is to have **one practical and/or cipher activity for each concept or idea** you want to explain.

We believe that all children learn better if they are able to physically engage in activities, with the activities being adapted if necessary to accommodate their physical abilities. The same is true for children with DME/2e and allowing them the opportunity to be physically involved in activities is very effective, especially if they display psychomotor overexcitability or the need to move or fidget significantly more than their peers.

We understand that all children love adventure and mystery but have found that children with DME/2e in particular seem to appreciate activities that have a definite element of mystery or novelty during therapy. These are activities that require problem solving, imagination and cognitive effort. This kind of activity does seem to be craved more by children with DME/2e than by those who would not be considered to have this profile.

Some examples of how to include practical and cipher activities in sessions

Example 1

At the start of the therapy process the therapist can explain to the child that there are two main categories (or strategies) they can use to help change how they feel, which are sensory- and thinking-based strategies. However, instead of telling the child what these are, the therapist can present them with different types of "secret code or cipher sheets" that all contain the same information on subcategories, such as "movement", "vision" and "sound", or "schedules" and "classifying problems" hidden within the codes or ciphers. The child can then decide which type of worksheets they would like to use, such as tap code, pigpen cipher, substitution cipher (e.g. numbers for letters) and proceed to decipher the words. If the child struggles to complete the sheets because of issues such as handwriting difficulties or having severe anxieties about writing, the therapist or parent can assist by writing down the letters the child decodes.

Example 2

A good way for a therapist to teach a child about using "movement" as a sensory strategy to help change how they feel is to invite them to engage in different types of movement activities during a session to practically illustrate the point. The therapist should present activities where each one represents one type of movement only. For example, one of the activities can be to jump on a mini trampoline, which represents the vertical and linear movement of going up and down. The therapist may ask the child to consider how they feel before and after jumping on the trampoline. The therapist may then present the child with a worksheet containing pictures of the movement activities presented in a column to the left of the page and descriptions of the movement types written down in random order to the right of the page. The child can then be asked to connect the movement/activity they have just done (in the left column), with the correct movement description in the right column, while also making a note of whether they liked or disliked that particular type of movement.

We have discovered it can sometimes help children with DME/2e when activities are deliberately presented incorrectly, with a high probability of not achieving a set goal, or where the outcome or message of an activity is delayed either to the end of a session or a follow up session. These strategies help to address their perfectionism, fear of failure, a fixed mindset and/or negative thought patterns that are impacting on their lives and activity participation. They also enjoy the process and seem to appreciate this "messing with their heads".

Some examples of designing unexpected or delayed outcomes

Deliberately presenting activities incorrectly

When a child with DME/2e has a love of maths, a sense of subtle humour or the ability to develop it, but also displays a fixed mindset, the therapist may choose to deliberately present some activities in the incorrect way. We always recommend therapists start sessions with some kind of visual schedule of the activities planned for the session. If the activities are numbered, therapists may choose to number them incorrectly such as −1 for activity one, 0 for activity two, 1 for activity three, 2 for activity four, and then 7.1 for activity five. The child will most assuredly notice this instantly and point out or ask why the numbering is incorrect. The therapist may respond with, "I was just joking to see if you would notice", or if it feels appropriate, ask the child why she thinks the numbering is incorrect without confirming or denying the child's answer is correct. This should all be done in good humour. We have found that most children with DME/2e will seem bemused and/or baffled, but even without further explanation, they seem to accept the imperfection and relax a bit more for the rest of the session.

Presenting activities with a high probability of not achieving a set goal

The following activity is helpful for children with DME/2e who have a love of art but who also display a fear of failure and/or perfectionism. These children often have extreme emotional reactions when situations do not go as they perceive they should or others do not act as they would like them to. The activity in itself is simple: you place a paper plate in a fully sealable salad spinner, add different coloured paints, close the lid and spin the plate a few times. The results are beautiful, but it is impossible to create the exact same painting twice.

Prior to a session, the therapist should make one of these paintings and allow it to dry fully. In the session itself, the therapist can show the child the painting and ask them to recreate the painting exactly, providing all the necessary materials. The child will undoubtedly mention it is not possible to recreate it exactly, but the therapist should encourage the child to try anyway. Once the child has made one painting, which may look similar but not 100% the same as the example, the therapist should ask the child a few questions such as whether the painting is beautiful or interesting (it almost always is!), whether theirs looks exactly the same as the example, etc. This can then lead into a discussion about how things may not always turn out the way we expect them to, but that the alternative outcome is not necessarily a bad one. The therapist can then link this concept to a particular situation where the child displays perfectionism that negatively impacts on their activity participation. Please also refer to Figure 6.2 for a visual representation of this activity.

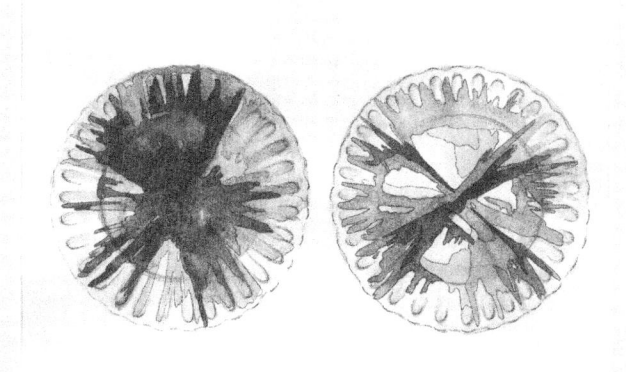

Figure 6.2 Salad spinner paintings.

Delaying the outcome or message of an activity

When a child with DME/2e struggles with negative thought patterns and associated negative self-talk, the therapist may plan to address this directly towards the latter part of the therapy process when it is more likely that a strong and trusting relationship has been established with the child. However, the therapist may introduce a related activity in a session a few weeks before the planned session. For example, we have found the "grass head" activity to be fun but with a powerful message regarding the impact of negative thought patterns and self-talk, if presented in the following way.

To create a grass head,[10] start by filling up a short stocking with grass seed followed by compost until you have a tennis ball sized shape. Tie it off, pinch the front of the head to make a nose and then hold the nose in place with an elastic band. Stick on some googly eyes and felt to make a mouth, and place it in a cup with the stocking tail dangling in the cup but without filling the cup with water.

The therapist should make one grass head before the session and explain to the child how to make one or demonstrate how to make one in the session itself. If the child struggles to make the grass head due to difficulties with organisation or fine motor skills, the therapist should assist the child as necessary as the goal of the activity is not to address these difficulties but to use the end product to explain the impact of positive and negative thought patterns and self-talk in a later session. Once the child has made the grass head, the therapist should instruct the child to take home both grass heads with strict instructions to only spray water onto one of the grass heads for the following two weeks – labelling the cup of the one that needs to be watered. The child will most probably ask what the point of the activity is and/or why they have to water only the one, but the therapist can respond by saying that they will discuss this in the next session and/or after at least two weeks.

After two weeks, the child should take the grass heads to the session in which the therapist plans to address thought patterns and related self-talk. If the child is unable to take the grass heads to the session, then they can take photos of the grass heads instead. If the child has only watered one of the grass heads, this grass head will have started to grow significantly more grass than the one that was not watered.

The therapist can use this as an analogy to demonstrate the concept or idea that whichever self-talk we use the most, just like the grass head that got watered the most, will "grow" more in our lives. So if we focus on positive self-talk, we will generally feel more regulated and confident in our abilities, which results in participating more easily in the activities that are important to us. However, if we focus more on negative self-talk, we will generally feel more dysregulated and doubtful of our abilities, which results in activity participation being more difficult than it should be. Please also refer to Figure. 6.3 for a visual representation of this activity.

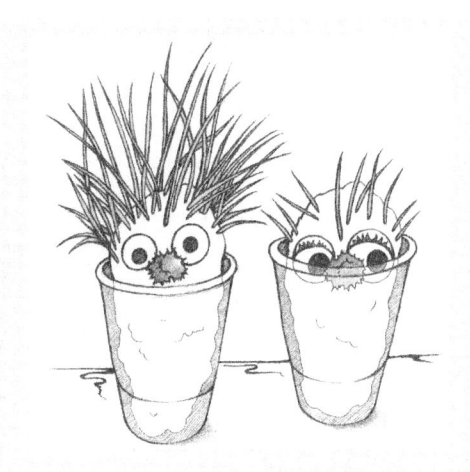

Figure 6.3 Grass heads.

Therapists may build up a bank of activities which they find meet these criteria and which they find work successfully with different children (as they will still be novel for each child). This is totally acceptable and will help therapists to standardise their own personal approach to therapy, which may save on preparation time in the long run. But we want to caution therapists against becoming too comfortable with their bank of activities and to always actively consider whether the activities they plan on using in sessions are suitable for a particular child considering their personality and preferences, or whether they may need to find some alternative ones.

Golden Nugget 9: Find the WOW and Super WOW Factors

The Cambridge Dictionary defines the word "wow"[11] as an exclamation, noun or verb. It is used to show surprise and sometimes pleasure (exclamation e.g. "*Wow*, did you see that?"), to describe a person or thing that is very successful, attractive or pleasant (noun e.g. "That song is just *wow!*") or to make someone feel great excitement or admiration (verb e.g. "He *wowed* the audience with his performance on stage").

In the DME-C approach, the WOW Factor is when therapists present sessions in such a way that children are "wowed" by it. Therapists can do this by tailoring sessions to cater to each child's individual likes and dislikes. This will mean the children will look forward to sessions, feel motivated to participate, engage with occupational therapy homework between sessions and get the most from therapy. The techniques and strategies they learn will help them manage their sensory processing differences and thought life, which influences their emotions more effectively in everyday life. In other words, by making sessions relevant to a child's individuality, the therapist is acknowledging the child's interests and this, by default, qualifies as finding the WOW Factor. By way of further explanation, we have given some examples of finding the WOW Factor below.

Some examples of finding the WOW Factor

Example 1

Sadie, a six-year-old child, is fascinated by dinosaurs. She has poor gross motor skills and is desperate to play hopscotch with her friends at school, but keeps tripping over her feet and almost always loses. Sadie now becomes embarrassed when she is asked to play, but instead says that she does not feel too well and would rather watch the others. One of her goals in therapy is to be able to complete a hopscotch course three times in a row without touching the lines of the squares. However, she is also initially shy and afraid to practise hopscotch in therapy. To help motivate her, the therapist suggests that the hopscotch course is a road into the jungle where the dinosaurs live, but the sides of the squares are volcanic ash which is harmful to dinosaurs, and therefore cannot be touched by any part of her feet as she hops through the course. Through using guided discovery questions as part of the CO-OP Approach™ the therapist assists Sadie to figure out ways of avoiding touching the volcanic ash. This pretend play addressed Sadie's imaginational overexcitability, and her shyness and reluctance soon diminishes as she stays engaged and focused on improving her hopping skills. Within six sessions Sadie manages to complete a hopscotch course three times successfully, and Sadie cannot be more pleased with herself!

Example 2

An eight-year-old child, Tristan, loves musical performances and shows. He also struggles with handwriting and has attended extra handwriting classes at school for almost a year with little improvement in the legibility of his writing.

When he starts with therapy and is told that he will need to complete some handwriting practice at home for five minutes every second day between sessions, he becomes oppositional. The therapist explores why he is reluctant to do the practice, and Tristan states he has completed multiple handwriting worksheets over the last year and that repeated practice of the alphabet has not helped so far. The therapist reassures him they will work at his pace, and he will only have to practise the letters they have done in a session, e.g. the "curly caterpillar letters" a, c, and o. To motivate Tristan to persist with the homework, the therapist prints off the lyrics of his favourite musical songs and instructs him to highlight all the words that start with a, c and o, and to then practise writing these words while only focussing on the correct formation of the first letters (and not the rest of the words initially). As therapy progresses, Tristan consistently does his OT homework, and his handwriting starts improving. Therapy also impacts his performance in other school related tasks. His mother sends the therapist a photo of a drawing he made and coloured in, stating, "I had to share Tristan's latest drawing with you! He has never drawn or coloured so neatly before!"

In using the DME-C approach, we have also discovered another layer to the WOW Factor that, if found, can have a significantly positive impact on other areas of the child's life beyond the therapy setting. We call this the "Super WOW Factor".

The Super WOW Factor revolves around **changing perspectives that create "aha" moments which lead to lasting change for the child**, either in the way they view their difficulties, or by identifying negative or unproductive thought patterns and changing their perspective on them. This means it is easier for them to be their true selves and/or participate in the activities they want to do. While creating aha moments is not exclusive to working with children with DME/2e, their perspectives often relate to the common characteristics identified in children who have high learning potential.

Finding the Super WOW Factor relies on having a non-judgemental approach to the child, affirming them for who they are and developing a good rapport. With this basis, unhelpful perspectives will come to the surface with time, and therapists can address them when they do. Doing this will require some creativity and "out of the box thinking" by the therapist and will differ from one therapist to the next depending on their personalities and the resources available to them, as well as the child's personality. Ultimately, the goal of the therapist is to change the child's perspective. So, instead of viewing a difficulty as a "weakness", it could be seen as a strength, and instead of viewing a unique characteristic as something to hide or be ashamed of, it could help them get closer to fulfilling a bigger plan or dream for their lives. By way of further explanation, we have given some examples and a case study of finding the Super WOW Factor below.

Some examples of finding the Super WOW Factor and how it can lead to lasting change for a child

Example 1

A nine-year-old boy called Dillan with high learning potential and an exceptional talent for playing musical instruments also has a severe sensitivity to sound, and, as a result, avoids going to musical performances even though he would very much like to. He feels confused that he can both "love" and "hate" music at the same time. The therapist works with Dillan to understand and manage his auditory sensitivity and encourages him to use some of the management strategies he is learning in therapy to help him go to a performance in his local town. Dillan decides to go with his mother and reports back to the therapist that overall he was able to cope. He also brings along his recorder to the next session and plays a piece of music for the therapist. Once he is finished, the therapist looks him in the eye and says, "Do you realise that your sensitivity to sound is what is helping you be a talented musician?" And "aha", the penny drops for Dillan. After this, he is determined to learn more about ways to manage his auditory sensitivity. His mother reports he seems invigorated to practise his recorder for longer times and is starting to talk about one day playing in the Royal Philharmonic Orchestra.

Example 2

Jess is an eleven-year-old girl with high learning potential and a talent for art who also has sensitivity to visually busy environments. She reports that she struggles to understand why she feels anxious in class but better on the playground during break times. During therapy, Jess realises she is bothered by all the visuals on the walls of the classroom, as she is "aware of everything". She starts developing some management strategies but now views this visual oversensitivity as a stumbling block. The therapist designs an activity where she invites Jess and her father (a builder who confesses Jess gets her talent for art from her mother's side of the family), who is attending the session, to write down all the colours they can see in a copy of Van Gogh's *Cafe Terrace at Night* painting in 30 seconds. Once they are done, they count the number of colours identified by each. Jess has identified four more colours than her dad, and the therapist asks her to discuss what the activity and the outcome mean to her. Jess responds that seeing fine detail in images can actually help her become a better artist or even an art historian one day. Jess realises that her "weakness" is actually a strength, and she is now talking about enrolling on an Arts Award* to pursue her passion for art with like-minded children. Aha!

Example 3: A case study

Children with HLP sometimes have interests outside the norm for their age which they pursue intensely and may make them come across as quirky, intense or strange to others. The children are often acutely aware of being different, and they may view this as a weakness or may have been led to believe that it is so by others. This was the case when an occupational therapist worked with an almost nine-year-old child with DME/2e called Katy who described herself as particularly "quirky" with regards to her way of viewing the world. For instance, her parents reported that she wrote "out of the box stories".

Katy was very aware she was different from her peers and in particular tried to hide her intelligence and quirkiness, sometimes suppressing her own expressions and feelings when amongst her peers in an attempt to fit in. The therapist decided to challenge Katy on this issue and gave her a poem to read called "Our Deepest Fear"[12] as part of her occupational therapy homework with the instruction to write down what it made her think of. In the following session, Katy shared what she thought about the poem, which was "... it makes me think that life isn't about being normal, like other kids. Life is about being yourself and letting your inner core hammer through everybody's minds so they can see who you really are". The therapist reported that this realisation helped Katy to accept herself for who she was and also motivated her to advocate for herself and find strategies to deal with her sensory processing differences.

Almost 18 months after therapy had ended, Katy's mother contacted the therapist to report she had been accepted into a prestigious performing arts state school for girls in London. What made this significant was that she was awarded one of only two places out of 250 applicants, which the mother credited in part to the family having worked with the therapist.

As part of the school's assessment process, the school advised that children should wear "comfortable clothes". On the morning of the assessment, Katy stated she wanted to stay in her pyjamas as it was her most comfortable clothes. The mother agreed as she understood the need for Katy to feel comfortable from a sensory perspective and herself. The mother stated, "She went completely comfortable in her own skin and, with an assessment consisting of movement and creativity and in her comfortable pyjamas, said she felt absolutely able to be her true self".

Although it is fairly easy to find the WOW factor in therapy, it may not always be possible to find the Super WOW Factor or Factors, as the child may not have unhelpful perspectives affecting how they view themselves or their difficulties. However, we still want to encourage therapists to continue creating a safe therapy space in case unhelpful perspectives surface, so therapists can address such thought patterns appropriately and creatively.

Golden Nugget 10: Foster a growth mindset

The terms "growth mindset" and "fixed mindset" are used to describe the underlying beliefs people have about their learning and intelligence.[13] It was first coined by Carol Dweck, Lewis and Virginia Eaton Professor of Psychology at Stanford University and the author of *Mindset: The New Psychology of Success*, after becoming interested in children's attitudes about failure and studying the behaviour of thousands of children.

Professor Dweck states,[14]

> We found that students' mindsets – how they perceive their abilities – played a key role in their motivation and achievement, and we found that if we changed students' mindsets, we could boost their achievement. More precisely, students who believed their intelligence could be developed (a growth mindset) outperformed those who believed their intelligence was fixed (a fixed mindset). And when students learned through a structured program that they could "grow their brains" and increase their intellectual abilities, they did better. Finally, we found that having children focus on the process that leads to learning (like hard work or trying new strategies) could foster a growth mindset and its benefits.

In her Ted Talk, Developing a Growth Mindset,[15] Professor Dweck further describes that children with a growth mindset understand their abilities can grow through their hard work. Their response to failure or error is therefore to process it deeply, learn from it (including accepting feedback) and correcting it. She links a growth mindset to the "power of yet". In other words, when children have setbacks, if they believe that they cannot do something yet and that they will be able to in the future, in other words "not yet", then they are more likely to put in the effort needed to learn that thing.

In contrast, Professor Dweck describes children with a fixed mindset as having the belief that their abilities and intellect are predestined and unable to improve. Their response to failure is to run away from it, resulting in no learning taking place. She links a fixed mindset to the "tyranny of now". In other words, when children have setbacks, if they are devastated because they not only believe they cannot do something at that time, but that they will not be able to do it in future either, they are less likely to put in the effort needed to learn that thing.

Professor Dweck gives some insightful guidelines on how to help children develop growth mindsets and refers to this as "building the bridge to yet". She emphasises that people should **praise or encourage children's effort, strategy** and **process**, and not just results.

Hundreds and perhaps thousands of people have adopted and written about the growth mindset philosophy, which is not just applicable to children, but to adults as well, and across various spheres of life (or activities of daily living), not just academic achievements. Below are some guidelines on developing a growth mindset, but this is by no means an exhaustive list and we encourage therapists to do further self-study into the topic.

Developing a growth mindset

- Praise wisely. When we praise children for their natural talent and intelligence, we reinforce that their abilities and intelligence are fixed. This leads to them giving up more easily after failure or makes them afraid to attempt tasks outside of their comfort zone. Instead, we should praise all children for the **effort** and focus they put in when engaged in tasks
- Raise (or approach) children for "yet" instead of "now". Within a learning context, the focus should be on the **process** of learning, development and improvement, instead of just getting good scores in tests
- Change children's mindsets directly by teaching them that if they are pushed out of their comfort zone when learning something new that is very hard, but they persevere, the neurons in their brains could form new stronger connections and over time they can become stronger
- When children experience setbacks, help them understand they cannot do something "yet". Difficulty just means "not yet". This creates confidence and helps them to develop greater persistence
- Encourage children to try **different strategies**. When children experience setbacks, it is not enough to tell them to just try harder, as they may repeat the same mistakes. Children should be encouraged to think of what they can do differently the next time they are faced with the problem
- Encourage children to tackle difficult tasks and assure them it is okay to make mistakes, as it is part of the learning process
- Encourage children to see new events or challenges as opportunities for learning and to value feedback, by actually praising them when they ask for feedback

A word of caution from Professor Dweck is to guard against a "false growth mindset",[16] which a colleague of hers in Australia, Susan Mackie, first identified. It is when adults claim to have a growth mindset, but their words and actions do not reflect it. A tell-tale indicator of this is when adults respond to children's mistakes as though they are problematic or harmful rather than helpful. This is likely to lead to children developing more of a fixed mindset about their intelligence. One way to help adults adopt a deeper and true growth mindset that will reflect in their attitudes towards children is to acknowledge we are all a mixture of fixed and growth mindsets, that we will probably always be, and that if we want to move closer to a growth mindset in our thoughts and practices, then we need to stay in touch with our fixed mindset thoughts and deeds.

How a growth mindset applies to the occupational therapy setting for children with DME/2e

Although the philosophy of growth mindset was originally developed in response to research into children's underlying beliefs about their learning and intelligence in an academic context, it is easy to see how the principles of fostering a growth mindset can be very helpful in the therapeutic setting.

Children with DME/2e with challenges relating to sensory processing, unhelpful thought patterns and self-regulation, perhaps more than their peers who are not considered to have DME/2e, may enter the therapeutic relationship with a fixed mindset about their intelligence and overall ability to learn, resulting in them avoiding challenging situations in therapy. They may enjoy learning about new concepts and strategies to help with their identified challenges but there is an underlying belief that they cannot "learn" how to manage these difficulties in real life, which acts as a potential barrier to implementing management strategies.

Fostering a growth mindset throughout the therapy process, and even afterwards, is of utmost importance. Learning how to do this is a continuous process, and we have found that it takes conscious effort as we often come across some of our own fixed mindsets. What we have found very helpful is to, firstly, constantly communicate to children that we believe in them and their ability to learn how to manage their needs in ways that work for them and that mistakes are okay since they are opportunities to learn. Secondly, model a growth mindset. The latter means being vulnerable when we make mistakes and modelling our response to failure.

An example of a therapist making a mistake and modelling a growth mindset

A therapist booked a day of administration into her diary, in order to catch up on paperwork, but forgot she had previously booked a child with DME/2e and his parent in for a double session on the same day using a different diary. The pair had travelled quite a distance for the appointment, but as they knocked on the door the therapist was shocked to see them. Instead of being courteous when she opened the clinic door, she blurted out "What are you doing here?". The parent explained they had an appointment, and the therapist had to apologise and state that she forgot. The parent was understandably upset and the therapist explained she could still see them as she did not have other sessions booked for the day. However, the therapist realised she did not feel regulated at that moment and that she would therefore not be able to give her full attention to the session. The therapist asked the pair whether they would mind waiting another half an hour. They were happy to do so as there was a coffee shop nearby, and they stated that they felt tired after the long car journey.

During the following half an hour, the therapist composed herself, using many of the calming sensory strategies she was teaching the child during the therapy process. When the session finally started, the therapist took full responsibility for forgetting the session and used it as an example of what she had learnt from her mistake. For one, it was to make sure that in future she only used one diary to book appointments! Secondly, the therapist could share with the child that her shock made her feel dysregulated, which led to her rude comment when she opened the door for them. While not totally acceptable, it was understandable, and the therapist modelled how to advocate for herself. Lastly, the therapist shared the sensory strategies she had used in the previous half an hour to help her calm down and feel more regulated.

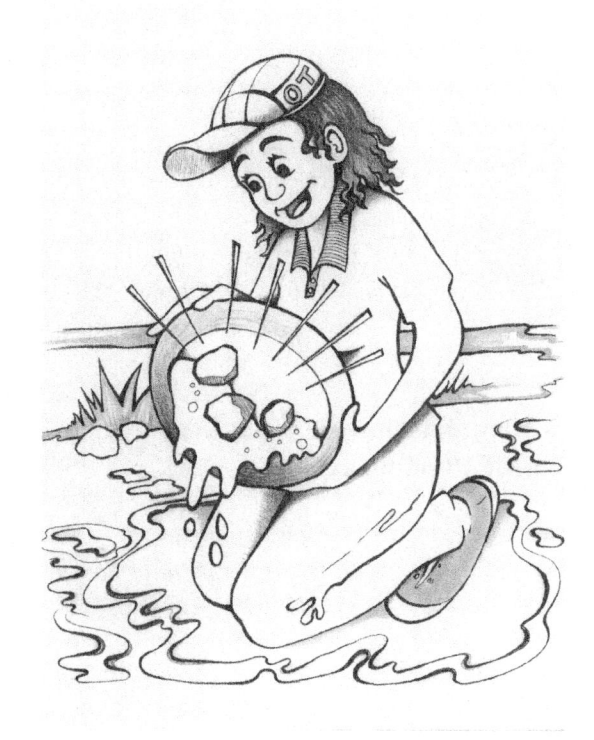

Conclusion

We trust therapists now have a clearer understanding of the 10 Golden Nuggets and how to apply them in their work with children with DME/2e regardless of their SEND. Not all of the Golden Nuggets will apply to every child, but we believe therapists will naturally gravitate to the ones that are the most relevant considering the particular child they are working with. Now that we have laid the foundation of the DME-C therapy approach, we can move onto Chapter 7 where we discuss the four walls or "4 Essential Components" to consider as part of therapy.

Notes

* Arts Award is a suite of arts-based qualifications for all young people aged 25 and under in the UK and managed by Trinity College London in Association with Arts Council England. Information at https://www.artsaward.org.uk/site/?id=2300.

References

1. Villanueva, S. A. & Huber, T. (2019) The issues in identifying twice exceptional students: A review of the literature. *International Journal of Development Research 09*.
2. Yates, D. (2022) *Parenting dual exceptional children: Supporting a child who has high learning potential and special educational needs and disabilities*. Jessica Kingsley Publishers.
3. Krausz, Lisa (2017) Understanding the Learning & Advocacy Needs of a Twice-Exceptional Student Through A Strengths-Based Lens: Review of the Literature. *Scholarship and Engagement in Education: Vol. 1: Iss. 1, Article 10*.
4. Cuncic, A. (2022, May 17) 'What is imposter syndrome? *Very Well Mind*. https://www.verywellmind.com/imposter-syndrome-and-social-anxiety-disorder-4156469.
5. Cox, L. K., (2023, March 28) Imposter Syndrome: 8 Ways to Deal With It Before it Hinders Your Success, Hubspot. Retrieved and adapted on April 12, 2023 from https://blog.hubspot.com/marketing/impostor-syndrome-tips.
6. Cambridge Dictionary. (n.d.) Boundary. In Dictionary.Cambridge.org. Retrieved on February 7, 2023 https://dictionary.cambridge.org/dictionary/english/boundary.
7. George, C. A., (2019, June 24). Setting effective boundaries with your gifted child or teen. *Christy George LMFT*. Retrieved on September 16, 2022 from https://www.christy-georgelmft.com/post/2019/06/24/set-effective-boundaries-with-your-gifted-child-or-teen.
8. Jacobsen, R. (n.d.) Teaching kids about boundaries. *Child Mind Institute*. Retrieved on April 21 2023 from https://childmind.org/article/teaching-kids-boundaries-empathy/.
9. Christy A. George, C. A., (24 June 2019, June 24). Setting effective boundaries with your gifted child or teen. Christy George LMFT. Retrieved on September 16, 2022 from https://www.christygeorgelmft.com/post/2019/06/24/set-effective-boundaries-with-your-gifted-child-or-teen.
10. Bunnings Warehouse. (2014,March 31) *How to make a grass head - DIY at Bunnings*. [Video] YouTube. https://www.youtube.com/watch?v=LguezfzXA00.
11. Cambridge Dictionary. (n.d.) Wow. In *Dictionary.Cambridge.org*. Retrieved on September 30, 2022 from https://dictionary.cambridge.org/dictionary/english/wow.
12. Williamson, M. (1992), *Our Deepest Fear*. in A Return to Love: Reflections on the Principles of A Course in Miracles. Harper Thorsens.
13. Mindset Works (n.d.) *Dr. Dweck's research into growth mindset changed education forever*, retrieved on October 13, 2022 from https://www.mindsetworks.com/science/.

14 Dweck, C. (2015, September 22) Carol Dweck Revisits the 'Growth Mindset'. *Education Week.* https://www.edweek.org/leadership/opinion-carol-dweck-revisits-the-growth-mindset/2015/09.
15 TED. (2014, October 9) *Developing a Growth Mindset* | Carol Dweck [Video]. YouTube. https://www.youtube.com/watch?v=hiiEeMN7vbQ.
16 Dweck, C. (2015, September 22) Carol Dweck Revisits the 'Growth Mindset'. *Education Week.* https://www.edweek.org/leadership/opinion-carol-dweck-revisits-the-growth-mindset/2015/09.

Chapter seven
The DME-C Approach's Four Walls
The 4 Essential Components

Introduction

In Chapter 6 we discussed the raw materials that make up the **foundation** of the DME-C therapy approach called the 10 Golden Nuggets, which concerns the **method** through which occupational therapists provide therapy.

In this chapter, we look more closely at the **four walls** of the DME-C therapy approach, called the "4 Essential Components", which are represented by the letters D, M, E and C. These essential components should be **addressed in any therapy provision with a child with DME/2e, sensory processing differences, unhelpful thought patterns and difficulties with emotional control or self-regulation**. We discuss the components individually but also demonstrate how they relate to or weave into one another. Once paediatric occupational therapists are aware of the components they need to consider in their therapy, they can draw on their own knowledge and experience to design activities that meet the requirements of these components.

We remind therapists that, although we have used the letters D, M, E and C for their similarity to **D**ual or **M**ultiple **E**xceptional **C**hildren to describe the 4 Essential Components, they must be combined with the 10 Golden Nuggets to make up the full DME-C therapy approach.

As occupational therapists read this chapter, they will see that the 4 Essential Components of (1) **D**iarise, (2) **M**anage transitions, (3) change the **E**nvironment and h**E**lp the senses and (4) **C**ommunicate are not novel concepts. In fact, they are part of the fundamental nature of occupational therapy training both pre- and post-qualification, a wider set of interventions as well as informal peer discussions, and it is therefore hard to pinpoint their exact origins. However, we have discovered the optimum strategies for the therapist's approach (10 Golden Nuggets) and the essential components (D, M, E and C) when providing therapy for children with DME/2e, and that, we believe, is novel. Please refer to Figure 7.1, The DME-C therapy approach's four walls: The 4 Essential Components, which provides a summary that can be printed for easy reference.

DOI: 10.4324/9781003334033-7

The DME-C therapy approach's four walls:
The 4 Essential Components

D: **D**iarise
M: **M**anage transitions
E: change the **E**nvironment and h**E**lp the senses
C: **C**ommunicate

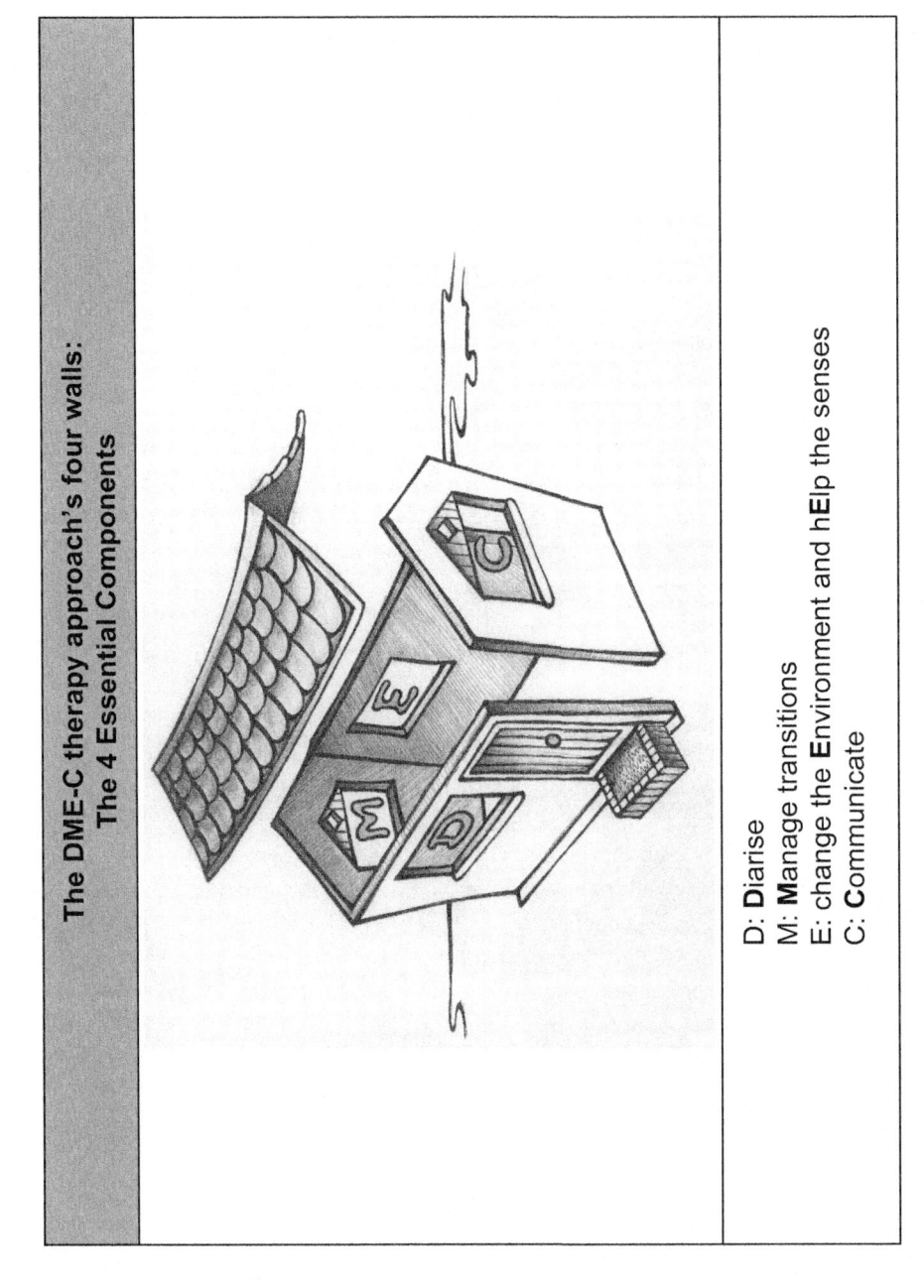

Figure 7.1 The DME-C therapy approach's four walls: The 4 Essential Components, M. Ferreira, R. Howell.

Copyright material from Mariza Ferreira and Rebecca Howell (2024),
Occupational Therapy for Children with DME or Twice Exceptionality, Routledge

Essential Component 1: Diarise

- Main aim: To help a child with DME/2e anticipate potentially stressful situations that could result in dysregulation and/or inappropriate behaviours, and devise a plan of action to deal with them effectively

When children with DME/2e and their parents or carers seek out occupational therapy, they often cite their main concerns as difficulties coping with their environment such as sensitivities to noise or visually busy places, an increased need for physical movement more than their peers and emotional dysregulation with associated extreme emotional outbursts that are out of context to the situations. Although they generally have a rough idea of what causes the children's difficulties (the triggers), they often need further explanation. Their understanding is often influenced by the accessibility and availability of information through the internet, which varies in accuracy and quality.

To diarise, in other words for the child to start keeping a diary or journal of when they struggle to cope with their physical environment and/or emotions and feelings, is a concept therapists know about and use regularly, but is not necessarily emphasised to the child in therapy. Working with a child with DME/2e and their parents or carers to diarise seems like a simple component, and this is probably the reason it is often undervalued. However, it is essential for children with DME/2e because it helps them to develop self-awareness which can be built on in therapy. It is very important to empower children, parents and carers to build this skill into the children's lives so they will be equipped to not only identify triggers at the time they work with an occupational therapist, but also in future after therapy has stopped and the triggers invariably change.

In many of the cases where therapists work with children with DME/2e, **sensory processing differences** and/or **negative thought patterns** act as triggers for their difficulties to participate and behave appropriately in relevant activities. This falls within the remit or scope of most paediatric occupational therapists. This does not, of course, include the full spectrum of triggers such as motor based triggers which were covered under the section "Developmental coordination disorder or DCD, including dyspraxia" in Chapter 4, or deep rooted trauma triggers associated with negative life experiences such as neglect and physical or emotional abuse. In cases of the latter, therapists should consider whether they have the necessary training and experience to address the child's issues or whether a referral to another suitable occupational therapist, psychologist or psychiatrist is necessary.

It is advisable to explain the two main types of triggers that impact on feelings and/or behaviour fairly early in the process when working with children with DME/2e and their parents. Using simple but relevant examples can help them easily understand and remember the types of triggers, which will help them towards increased self-awareness and self-management. For example, if a child and their parent are late for their first therapy session because of heavy traffic on the way to the clinic, they may feel flustered and anxious when they arrive for their session. After the therapist reassures them, the therapist can start explaining there are two main types of triggers that can influence how they feel. The first type is from the **sensory environment,** e.g. the volume from the car radio possibly being too loud and causing a person to feel irritated, and the second is from a person's **thought environment,** e.g. the thought that they were going to be late and possibly miss their session, which caused them worry and anxiety.

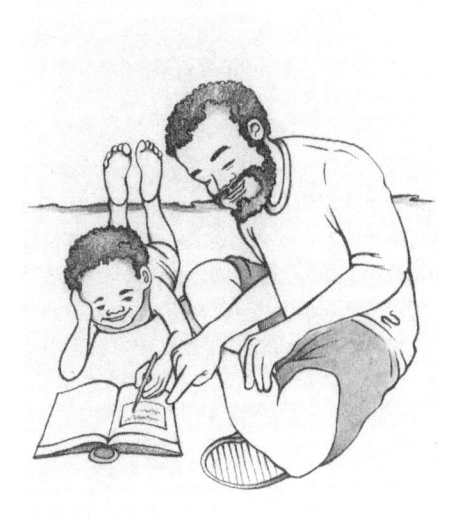

In addition, the therapist may proceed to explain that addressing or "tackling" negative and unhelpful sensory- and thought-based issues will in fact require using positive and helpful sensory- and/or thought-based strategies. However, the child will first need to figure out what their specific triggers are.

Keeping a diary is a systematic way to figure out a child's specific triggers, but it is advisable that the occupational therapist only encourages the child to start keeping a diary after a few sessions have been completed and the child has started to develop a language to describe their feelings (see "Essential Component 4: Communication"). Occupational therapists may coach the child with DME/2e and their parents to keep a diary of the main activities they engaged in on a particular day, and whether they felt calm, ready or "up to the task" in each particular activity or not. In other words, they diarise whether they could meet the occupational and/or self-regulatory demands of that particular activity or not. With regards to the activities where the child did not "feel up to the task", they should be encouraged to try and name or describe their feelings during the particular activities (if they are able). For example, being tired, sad, bored, anxious or angry. Furthermore, they should try and identify the behaviours they displayed, such as being unable to concentrate, argumentative, lashing out at others and screaming. At this point, the child and their parents should not attempt to analyse their feelings or behaviours, as this will be done with the therapist during therapy sessions. Some questions the therapist can use to assist in explaining how to keep a diary are as follow:

1. What was the activity?
2. How did you feel during the activity?
3. Did you feel up to the task or not?
4. How did you react during the activity, in other words what behaviours did you display?

It is a good idea to ask the child with DME/2e to keep a diary or journal for three to four days and to choose days that are different. For example, they can log their feelings and associated behaviours for a school day or home school day, a day over the weekend, a non-typical day such as when they go on a school trip and, if relevant, a day during the school holidays. It is important they log this physically in writing or on a computer and, where possible, to do this together with a parent or carer at the end of each day. Doing so will make it easier to identify triggers when discussing it with the therapist. The child can decide to use their own diary if they fully understand the task expectations, or therapists can supply the child with templates, either self-made or from existing professional programmes. As a side note, if the child has particular difficulties with handwriting and/or refuses to write or type, it could be done by a parent as the aim in this instance is not to improve the child's handwriting but to identify triggers.

During the therapy session where the occupational therapist and child with DME/2e review the diary they have kept, the therapist should help the child analyse the reasons they felt up to the task (regulated/correct arousal level) during certain activities, and identify the sensory- and/or thought-based (or other) triggers when they did not. This can be done by asking prompting questions such as:

1. Do you have any idea why you felt the way you did?
2. Was the room or area you were in very busy or noisy?
3. Did someone say something that made you feel upset?
4. Was there a change in the circumstances?
5. Did you enjoy the activity?
6. Did you feel the activity challenged you enough?
7. Did you feel bored during the activity?

It is important to spend enough time with the child with DME/2e reviewing the activities in the diary and to keep asking prompting questions and/or suggest possible reasons (triggers) for the feelings and behaviours the child had. This way the child will begin to understand which triggers were sensory and/or thought-based and which ones were rooted in something else. For example, a child may be able to tell the therapist they feel overwhelmed in certain environments such as noisy food halls and therefore become argumentative with their peers, but at other times they may just describe a physical awareness such as always getting a headache when in the hall. The therapist can then help the child make the link between their feelings and/or behaviours and the "sensory-based trigger" of auditory sensitivity or over-responsiveness (if the therapist has already established this during the assessment process prior to therapy). Similarly, if the child describes that they were in a quiet classroom but the work they had to do was too easy so they did not see the point of doing it and subsequently got told off by their teacher, the therapist can help them make the link between their feelings and/or behaviours and the "thought-based trigger" of "not seeing the point" leading to avoidance of work.

Once a child with DME/2e and their parents have a clearer understanding of the types of situations in which they are likely to feel dysregulated or not up to the task, whether because of sensory- or thought-based (or other) triggers, it will become easier for them to anticipate various stressful situations. This means they can plan ahead to use effective management strategies in each. As is life, it is not always possible to anticipate all stressful situations beforehand, but a child being more self-aware and knowing which management strategies work for them can help them to employ the strategies and feel regulated more quickly when they experience unexpected stressful situations (see "Essential Component 3, E: change the Environment and hElp the senses").

> **Two examples of children with DME/2e who used a diary to identify triggers**
>
> **Example 1: Sensory-based triggers**
>
> Timmy was a six-year-old child with high learning potential and severe auditory and tactile sensitivity. He loved science and wanted to go to the science museum in London with his mother. However, they had to go by train and the underground tube, which was a journey he did not feel up to as he found it too overwhelming. He was also afraid of facing the crowds at the museum itself. The occupational therapist worked with Timmy to use a diary to start identifying situations in which he felt comfortable and those in which he did not and therefore avoided.
>
> Once Timmy was able to understand how his auditory and tactile sensitivities were causing him to avoid activities he was keen to do, he took the reins with devising strategies to manage his difficulties. Soon after, his mother reported,
>
> Last Thursday we went to the science museum in London. It was a really lovely outing and our first day trip to London to visit a museum. Timmy enjoyed the museum very much. As well as visiting areas that interested him and trying an interactive task, he enjoyed a 3D film called *Under the Sea*. This was also our first cinema experience. We sat close to the exit, and he knew we could leave at any time if he needed to. I thought it was quite loud and full-on with all the colour, images and 3D, but he put on the 3D glasses and sat still throughout. He said the hardest part of the day was the travel - train and underground each way. We took our time and avoided the rush hours. There was an unpleasant screeching noise on the underground on the way back (wheels against the tracks as happens sometimes) and the man sitting next to me actually put his fingers in his ears, but I did not comment, and Timmy did not respond at all.
>
> **Example 2: Sensory- and thought-based triggers**
>
> Savannah was an eight-year-old girl with high learning potential, strong leadership qualities combined with a sense of right and wrong or "how things should be done", and particularly artistic and creative. She also displayed increased sensory seeking behaviour with regards to movement as opposed to her peers and auditory sensitivity.

Savannah started seeing an occupational therapist with the main concerns being that she was struggling with her sensory issues and managing her emotions. This impacted on her family life as she would often lash out at her siblings and damage furniture when feeling upset and dysregulated. Savannah would always feel very embarrassed after such episodes and was highly motivated to improve her self-awareness and develop effective strategies to help her cope. Following the end of occupational therapy, her parents reported,

In the sessions themselves, Savannah was given the time and space to practise strategies, to recognise trigger points and the indicators of escalating emotions. She still has regular challenges with her emotions, of course, but she now has insights and strategies that work.

Essential Component 2: Manage transitions

- Main aim: To help a child with DME/2e reduce anxiety that is related to transitions

Transition means to "change from one form or type to another, or the process by which this happens",[1] or in other words to change or move from one activity, environment, state, subject or situation to another.

It is well known that children with sensory processing differences generally struggle with transitions, and the same goes for children with DME/2e with sensory processing differences. This is because they fear or are anxious about the "unknown" sensory elements and other demands of the next activity, environment or situation. Children with DME/2e also have a tendency to "overthink" situations and/or expect the worst (imaginational overexcitability), so their anxiety levels may be palpable when it comes to transitioning or masked very well through delay tactics, such as a sudden interest to revisit topics discussed in a session when it is nearing the end.

Occupational therapists can easily help children with DME/2e and their parents learn how to manage transitions, which has the potential to significantly reduce their related-anxiety and avoidance behaviours over time. This can be done through:

1. Using strategies covertly* during therapy sessions, which is helpful for parents attending sessions to observe in order to better understand how to support their child with transitions
2. Purposefully exploring management strategies with children in order to find the ones that work best for them.

Some strategies we have found effective in therapy are listed below but therapists may use and develop additional strategies depending on the particular preferences of the child with DME/2e they are working with.

Using managing transitions strategies covertly in therapy

1. Using visual schedules to demonstrate session progression

In most cases, we recommend therapists have some sort of visual schedule ready at the start of therapy sessions, which is discussed with the child so they know what to expect in the sessions. The session activities and discussions may not always go to plan as a child may want to spend more time on a particular topic and less on another. It is therefore important to discuss with the child that it is a plan only and things may change, but this is okay as the sessions are not meant to be rigid.

Visual schedules may be on a blackboard, white board, paper, etc. and contain writing, pictures or a combination of both. Tailoring visual schedules to reflect the particular interests of a child with DME/2e is a fun way to get them interested and engaged while at the same time reducing their anxiety about the sessions. The child may also choose to wipe out activities once completed, draw a line through them, etc.

Below are some examples of visual schedules that have been used effectively in sessions. Figure 7.2 is a visual schedule with session progression represented by a battery circuit, which was used with a child with DME/2e who had a particular interest in how batteries work. Figure 7.3 is a visual schedule with session progression indicated by a road between activities for a five-year-old child with DME/2e who had a love for cars.

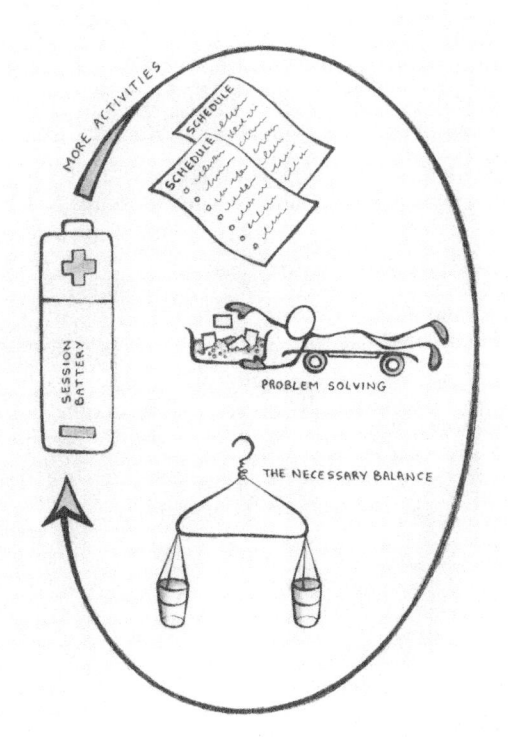

Figure 7.2 A visual schedule with therapy session progression represented by a battery circuit.

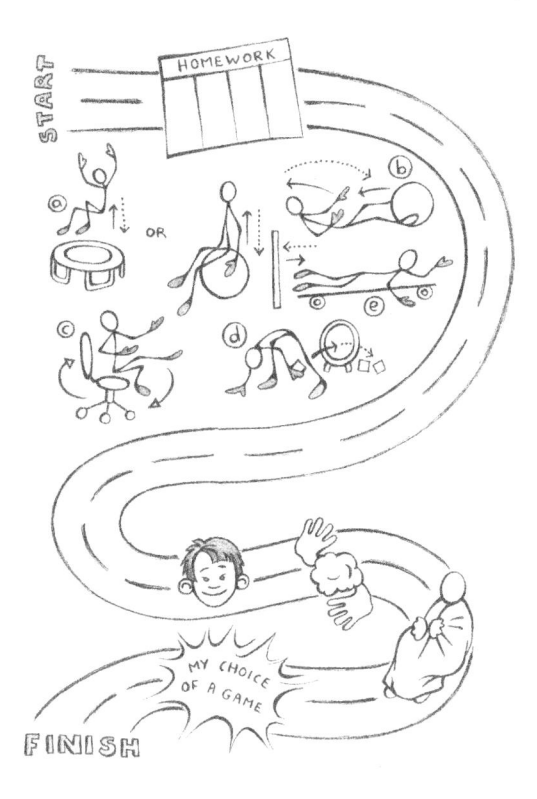

Figure 7.3 A visual schedule with therapy session progression indicated by a road between activities.

Although visual schedules are very effective in most cases to help manage transitions, there are rare occasions when they may have the opposite effect. An example of this is when a child has pathological demand avoidance (PDA) and feels totally overwhelmed by the "demands" listed on the schedule. Therapists should be aware of this possibility and explore alternative ways to help the child successfully manage transitions.

PDA is a profile on the autism spectrum involving resisting and avoiding everyday demands and a need for control driven by anxiety. It has a significant impact on an individual's everyday life and wellbeing. Currently it is not recognised as a formal standalone condition.[2]

2. **Discussing the next activity before the current one is finished**

This strategy is exactly what it says on the tin. Therapists may find that children initially struggle to engage in the first activity at the start of sessions, but when they start taking part, they can generally move easily from one activity to the next using the visual schedule as a guide. However, as they near the end of sessions, they may again have difficulty finishing and leaving the sessions. Therapists can deal with this by initiating conversations about what the child and their parents are planning to do after the session. For instance, if it happens to be near lunch time, the therapist can ask the child and his parents if they are planning to go for lunch after the session. If so, this could lead to a discussion about where they are planning to go and what they are likely to eat, and, if necessary, this could further develop into discussing coping strategies in case the restaurant or cafe happens to be busy, etc. This way the therapist is helping the child to transition out of the current environment and into the next one with less anxiety.

Purposefully exploring managing transitions strategies with a child with DME/2e

1. **Devising daily or weekly schedules**

It is advisable to set aside allocated time in therapy to discuss keeping a daily or weekly schedule as a strategy to help children with DME/2e manage transition related anxiety. Keeping a schedule of planned activities for the next day or week is beneficial because it allows a child the opportunity to anticipate potentially stressful situations and therefore plan ahead which sensory- and/or thought-based strategies they could use to help them cope. It can also empower the parent to advocate for their child with relevant teachers and other adults.

Whether the child chooses a daily or weekly schedule, it should ideally only contain the main activities for a particular day and especially activities that are out of the ordinary, e.g. a sports day at school, trip to the local zoo or a birthday party. Schedules work best if the child and parent or caregiver discuss the day's activities the night before, although discussing an activity which is a few days in advance (as in the case of a weekly schedule) can help the child and their parents make the necessary preparations. We do want to caution against rigid schedules that are set minute by minute or hour by hour, which do not allow for flexibility. This is because unforeseen circumstances and a resulting failure to keep to the schedule will increase the anxiety of a child with DME/2e who has perfectionist tendencies.

2. **Exploring specific transition activities**

When a therapist and a child with DME/2e have identified that they struggle with smaller scale transitions, such as moving from one lesson in school to the next, they can explore using specific short transition activities, such as having a two minute break between lessons during which they play with therapy putty, taking a quick walk down the school corridor and/or doing some exercises such as star jumps. These activities need to be chosen by the child to ensure they are appropriate and also communicated and agreed upon with the classroom teacher and/or SENDCO (special education needs and disabilities coordinator) at the school.

Therapists should also be aware that although "manage transitions" mainly refers to general or everyday transitions that children may experience, this can also refer to larger scale transitions or life events children with DME/2e may have particular difficulty coping with.

Examples of this are moving from one school phase to the next or moving up a year. In these situations, therapists can play a supportive role by providing a listening ear, addressing perceptions, encouraging the child to develop suitable coping and problem-solving strategies and suggesting additional professional support where necessary.

Essential Component 3: change the Environment and hElp the senses

- Main aim: To assist a child with DME/2e to develop increased self-awareness of how their sensory and thought environments affect their feelings and behaviours; and the principles of developing their own effective coping strategies

"change the Environment and hElp the senses" is focussed on teaching children with DME/2e the **underlying concepts and principles** of:

1. Identifying their own sensory needs and thought processes impacting on modulation, self-regulation and activity participation (feelings and behaviours)
2. Developing effective coping strategies for related challenges

Therapists will do well to remember that addressing a child with DME/2e's sensory environment means they are addressing the sensual and/or psychomotor overexcitabilities (see Chapters 2 and 5) impacting on the child's activity participation. In addition, addressing their thought environment means therapists are addressing the emotional, imaginational and, to an extent, the intellectual overexcitabilities (see Chapter 2) that have a negative impact.

Therapists will most likely, depending on their training, background and experience of working with children, be familiar with ways to help children develop increased self-awareness and coping strategies. However, when working with children with DME/2e, it is important they make a conscious effort to meet these children on their cognitive level (their "need to know" or intellectual overexcitability) as required. In other words, therapists may only need to explain how the body's sensory systems and the brain's basic thought patterns work and/or impact on a person's feelings and behaviours in a simplistic way, or they may need to go into a lot more depth on the subjects to satisfy the child's curiosity.

When considering a child's sensory environment, some will find it adequate to know that "certain movements can make me feel unwell and agitated", such as going on a roller coaster ride (increased self-awareness). Equally some will find it adequate to know that "certain movements can help change how I feel", such as jumping on a mini trampoline to help them feel more alert for schoolwork, or to "reset" when they are upset (coping strategy). Other children, and often their parents or carers, may find it fascinating to understand the mechanics or physiology of the vestibular system and therefore why the roller coaster or trampoline can have a particular effect on a person.

140 *The DME-C Approach's Four Walls*

Similarly, when considering a child's thought environment, some children will be satisfied with the explanation that ongoing and excessive negative thoughts about themselves and/or situations can have an overall impact on their mental and physical health.[3] However, others will want to explore the chain reaction that occurs when the amygdala, or emotional brain which produces the fight, flight or freeze response, perceives a "threat" which triggers the release of stress hormones that are responsible for elevated heart rate and blood pressure affecting mental and physical health over time.[4] These more in-depth discussions are generally very stimulating, but should they take up too large a part of a therapy session (which is rare), therapists can encourage the child and his parents to do further self-study on the topic.

"change the Environment and hElp the senses" by nature makes up a large part of the therapy process and because therapy generally progresses at an accelerated pace with children with DME/2e, instead of switching often between the difficulties being addressed, we suggest to first address the child's sensory environment and then their thought environment. However, there may be occasions when therapists feel it is more appropriate and/or urgent to first address the child's thought environment. With regards to addressing both environments, therapists may find it helpful to follow the "**S-TE-DD-R**" guidelines (similar to the word "**steadier**" in sound) which only has slight variations in its implementation as discussed below. S-TE-DD-R represents:

Subdivide ⇒ **T**each & **E**xperience / **E**xplore ⇒ **D**iscuss & **D**iscover ⇒ **R**emember

---

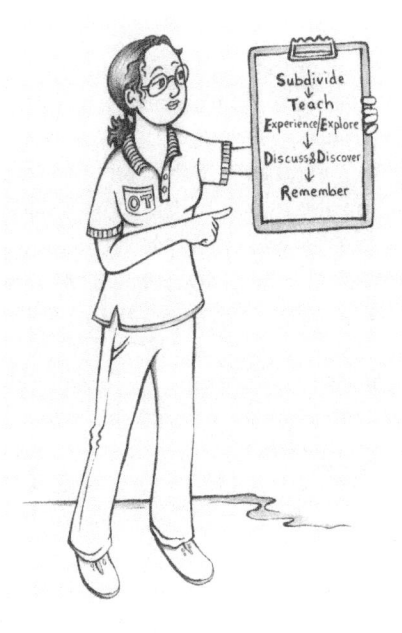

Figure 7.4 S-TE-DD-R: Subdivide - Teach & Experience/Explore - Discuss & Discover - Remember.

Subdivide

Subdivide, or identify, each sensory system into its various types of stimuli and the thought patterns that are influencing the child with DME/2e's modulation, emotional wellbeing, self-regulation and activity participation. In identifying thought patterns, it is important to keep in mind the common characteristics of children with HLP, Dabrowski's overexcitabilities and asynchronous development. Where possible, devise one activity to explain each type of sensory stimuli and thought pattern, although a combination of activities is often required to explain a thought pattern or combination of thought patterns. When it is not possible to physically engage in an activity, plan on using in-depth discussion aided by pictures, objects, analogies, metaphors, famous quotes, etc. to explain the types of stimuli or thought patterns.

Teach and Experience/Explore

Directly **teach** the child with DME/2e there are different types of sensory stimuli related to a specific sensory system and thought patterns that can influence how they feel and behave. Give the child the opportunity to **experience or explore** how each type of stimuli and (identified) thought pattern affects them by presenting activities for each by way of illustration and/or using in-depth discussion as necessary. This will help them develop increased self-awareness with regards to their sensory and thought environments.

Discuss and Discover

Discuss with the child their natural reaction to each type of sensory stimuli, regardless of whether this is negative or positive. For negative responses that impact activity participation, help the child **discover** suitable coping strategies by teaching the **sensory-**related discover principles of change the Environment and hElp the senses, which are:

- **Change** the physical environment with its sensory elements
- **Help** the sensory system that is "struggling" by using the same sensory system (or sense) but in a different way
- **Help** the sensory system that is "struggling" by activating another sensory system (or sense)

See "Addressing the child with DME/2e's sensory environment" for examples of the above.

Similarly, if the child is motivated to address certain thought patterns, the therapist should help the child **discover** suitable coping strategies by teaching the **thought**-related discover principles of change the Environment and hElp the senses which are:

- **Change** the unhelpful thought patterns in the thought environment
- **Help** the thought patterns that are "struggling" by activating their opposites

See "Addressing the child with DME/2e's thought environment" for examples of the above.

Remember

To help the child keep track of and **remember** their coping strategies and the related discover principles, ensure there is a physical reminder by providing them with a written summary of the key points covered in a session, any worksheets they have completed in sessions and/or homework they can complete between sessions. Encourage the child to keep all of these in a file for later reference.

Addressing the child with DME/2e's sensory environment

Table 7.1 shows the kinds of activities that can be used to illustrate different types of sensory stimuli.[5] Following the table, there is a practical example of how to achieve **S-TE-DD-R** with regards to the auditory system at the end of this section. We are aware that therapists may label the types of stimuli slightly differently, and they can continue to do so. We also encourage therapists to consider how they can use and adapt their existing and other mainstream activities to aid children's understanding in these areas.

Table 7.1 Sensory Environment: Types of Stimuli and Example Activities to Illustrate

Sensory Environment: Types of Stimuli and Example Activities to Illustrate		
Sensory System	Types of Sensory Stimuli	Basic Activities and Discussions to Illustrate Sensory Stimuli
Vestibular and proprioceptive systems	Movement types and body positions • Linear	Jump on a mini trampoline, or bounce on a therapy ball. Lie prone on a scooter board, scoot forward by kicking away from a wall and then move back in the same direction by pushing away from the opposite wall with your body facing the same direction throughout the activity.
	• Rotational	Spin round while standing or spin on a swivel chair.
	• Inversion	Whilst in an upside down position, throw bean bags to a hula hoop target through the legs.
	Load the joints (or heavy work) • Using gravity & • Adding weight	Lie on your back and move your hands and feet up simultaneously to touch in the middle. Then move a medium-sized ball from your feet to your hands and over your head. Reverse the movement.
	Movement and load the joints (combined)	Jump onto a large beanbag and/or discuss the effects of jumping onto a large beanbag or soft sofa.
Tactile system	Hands • Resistive materials • Different textures	Play with therapy putty and blue tac.

(Continued)

Table 7.1 (Continued)

Sensory Environment: Types of Stimuli and Example Activities to Illustrate		
Sensory System	Types of Sensory Stimuli	Basic Activities and Discussions to Illustrate Sensory Stimuli
	Face • Temperature	Splash face with warm or cold water, or discuss the effects of doing this.
	Body	Wrap yourself in a favourite blanket.
Oral (and olfactory) sensory systems	Deep breathing • In through nose • Out through mouth	Play adapted "noughts and crosses" by using straws to suck up and hold in place laminated paper shapes (representing the noughts and crosses) before placing them on a large grid made by ropes or sticking down tape on the floor (to illustrate the importance of deep breathing in although we are aware in reality this should be done through the nose). Please also refer to Figure 7.5 for a visual representation of this activity. Play with a floating ball toy (to illustrate the importance of deep breathing out through the mouth).
	Talking	Discuss the benefits of talking to a trusted adult about emotions.
	Food and drinks • The four T's	Discuss the **four T's** of food and drinks: textures, taste, thickness and temperature.
	Note regarding smelling of different fragrances:	Only discuss and/or experience (such as having a flannel sprinkled with a favourite fragrance, e.g. lavender drops) if the child mentions this in therapy. This is because odours or smells can have strong negative emotions for specific individuals, which can play a significant role in contributing to post traumatic stress disorder.[a]
Visual system	Colours • bright • dull	Discuss colours with the aid of small felt squares of different colours and colour depth.
	Distractions • many • few	Discuss distractions with the aid of pictures of a tidy and messy room.
	Light • natural • artificial	Discuss light by drawing attention to the effect of the ceiling (artificial) light in the therapy clinic and going outside to discuss the effect of natural light.

(Continued)

Table 7.1 (Continued)

Sensory Environment: Types of Stimuli and Example Activities to Illustrate		
Sensory System	Types of Sensory Stimuli	Basic Activities and Discussions to Illustrate Sensory Stimuli
	Artificial light • still • moving	Have a fibre optic light and small disco ball light to hand. Discuss the effect of each.
	Reading	Discuss reading as a strategy to help with self-regulation.
Auditory system	Type of environment • quiet • background noise	Discuss the effect of being in a quiet area vs. one with background noise.
	Non-human sounds • nature sounds • white noise	Use a music streaming service to listen to nature sounds and white noise, and discuss the effect of each.
	Volume of sound • loud • soft	Use a music streaming service to listen to a preferred song at various volume levels and discuss its effects, if any.
	Preferred music	Use a music streaming service to listen to a preferred song or music composition and discuss its effect. Listen to any other random song or music composition to discuss its effect and whether the child likes it.

[a] Stierwalt, S. (2020, June 29) Why do smells trigger memories? *Scientific American.* https://www.scientificamerican.com/article/why-do-smells-trigger-memories1/.

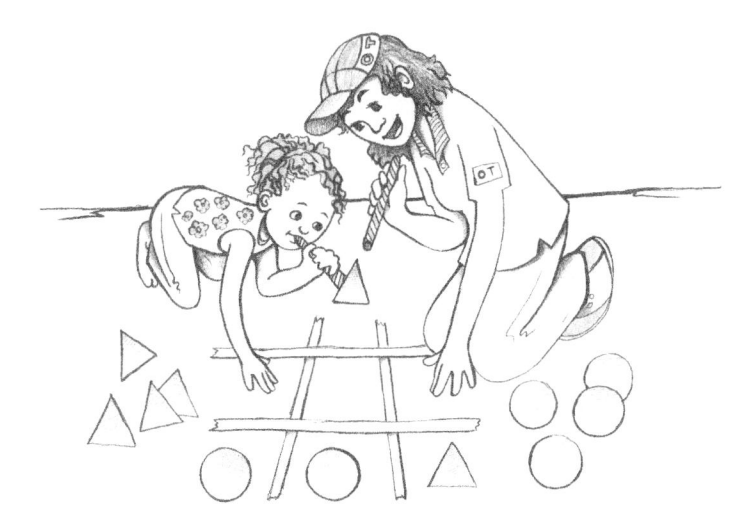

Figure 7.5 Adapted noughts and crosses.

An example of how to use S-TE-DD-R for the auditory system

When addressing the auditory system, it can be subdivided into different types of sensory stimuli, such as a quiet environment vs. one with background noise, nature sounds vs. white noise, the volume of sound and music the child prefers.

To teach each type of stimulus, the therapist should use a combination of discussions and activities. For example, the therapist can lead a discussion on how the child feels or reacts in a quiet environment, such as the quiet therapy clinic as opposed to when they go to a noisy party. The therapist can also use a digital music streaming service to listen to one of the child's favourite songs. They can then explore the child's reaction to it (always positive!) and how playing it at different volume levels affects them. Certain volume levels or changing volume levels may make them feel uncomfortable with the potential to dysregulate or not. Similarly, the therapist and child can explore listening to nature sounds and white noise and discuss their effects on the child.

When the child has a negative reaction in the session, or identifies that they generally have a negative reaction to one or all of the types of auditory stimuli, the therapist can encourage the child to think of specific situations where they may need to develop coping strategies. For example, if the child identifies that they struggle to do their homework at the dinner table with a noisy younger sibling next to them, then the therapist and child can discuss the "discover" principles of addressing it. Ways of **changing the physical environment** may include doing homework at the dinner table whilst wearing ear defenders and/or at a table in their bedroom as opposed to the dinner table. Ways of **helping the auditory system that is struggling by using the same auditory system in a different way** may include listening to their favourite music either before or whilst doing homework. And ways of **helping the auditory system that is struggling by**

activating another sensory system may include doing some seated heavy work (proprioceptive) activities, such as chair push ups, whilst doing homework.

Lastly, the therapist should provide the child with a written summary of the key elements explored during the session as well as an occupational therapy homework worksheet to identify at least one auditory strategy to help change how the child feels in a particularly stressful situation. The therapist should also make sure they discuss the homework at the start of the next session. Figure 7.6 an example of a session summary sheet. Please note it is an extract only, as generally other sensory systems would also have been covered in the session, such as the gustatory/oral and visual sensory systems.

Figure 7.6 An extract of a session summary sheet with related occupational therapy homework for sensory environment.

An extract of a session summary sheet with related occupational therapy homework
Child: **Date of session:**
Session number: **Venue:**
Persons present:

Today we explored how:

- Sounds and listening to things can influence how we feel. You probably realised that you like or don't like:
  - Working in a quiet environment or one with background noise.
  - Nature sounds and/or white noise.
  - Sounds that are loud or high in volume, and soft or low in volume.
- Listening to our favourite music and songs helps change how we feel.

Today we learnt that:

- We need to consider the impact of sound from our environment on how we feel, and that we can change how we feel if needed by:
  - Changing our environment, such as wearing noise cancelling headphones when doing homework or doing homework in a quieter space.
  - Helping our auditory (hearing) system that is struggling by using it in a different way, such as listening to our favourite music before we do homework.
  - Helping our auditory (hearing) system that is struggling by also activating another sensory system, such as doing chair push ups whilst we are doing our homework (proprioception or heavy work).

The OT homework to complete before the next session:
Use the worksheet: **These are my auditory- or hearing-related strategies to help me change how I feel**. In the week ahead, explore listening to different types of sounds like we did in the session, and identify at least one type of sound, or new song, to help change how you feel.

Addressing the child with DME/2e's thought environment

Table 7.2 shows the kinds of activities therapists can use to help children with DME/2e explore common types of thought patterns. The table is followed by a practical example of how to achieve **S-TE-DD-R** with regards to negative thought patterns expressed as being critical of self and inner dialogue or negative self-talk at the end of this section. As with addressing the child with DME/2e's sensory environment, we acknowledge therapists may label types of thought patterns differently to us, and they can continue to do so. We also encourage therapists to consider how they can use and adapt their existing and other mainstream activities to aid children's understanding in these areas.

Table 7.2 Thought Environment: Common Types of Thought Patterns and Suggested Exploration Activities

Thought Environment: Common Types of Thought Patterns and Suggested Exploration Activities	
Thought Pattern	Basic Activities and Discussions to Illustrate Thought Patterns
Perfectionism, expressed as: Fear of failure	Design activities with unexpected or delayed outcomes (see Chapter 6, Golden Nugget 8): • Deliberately present activities incorrectly, e.g. odd numbering of visual schedule activities • Present activities with a high probability of not achieving a set goal, e.g. "paper plate painting" using a salad spinner
Self-imposed high (and often unachievable) standards	As part of occupational therapy homework, ask the child to explore what they think about famous quotes related to perfectionism and discuss in a follow up session, e.g. "Perfection is the enemy of progress" by Winston Churchill.
Critical of self, with negative self-talk	See "negative thought patterns" below.
Emotional outbursts	See "concern with justice and fairness" below.
Negative thought patterns, expressed as: Critical of self or self-judgement	Ask the child how they would encourage or what kind words they would use to help a friend going through a similar difficult situation. Then encourage the child to "be their own best friend", and say those things to themselves in future.
Inner dialogue, often negative self-talk	Design activities with unexpected or delayed outcomes (see Chapter 6, Golden Nugget 8): • Grass head activity aided by discussion that, just like the grass head that got watered grew the most grass, the self-talk we use the most will have the most significant impact in our lives Prepare a worksheet with the words "negative self-talk" and "positive self-talk" written on it, and add related pictures and statements in random positions on the sheet, e.g. • Picture of a sunny sky • Picture of a cloudy sky • "Makes me doubt my ability to do things and reach my full potential" • "Helps me to feel confident in myself" • "The pessimistic voice in my head" • "The optimistic voice in my head" • "Always looks on the dark side" • "Robs me of my self confidence" • "The sunny voice in my head" • "The cloudy voice in my head" • "Always looks on the bright side" • "Helps me believe in my ability to do things and reach my full potential" Present the sheet to the child and ask them to connect the words to their corresponding pictures and statements. Discuss the two types of thinking with the child and which one they think they use the most. (A parent or carer's non-judgmental input can also be helpful in this regard, as some children may not initially be totally forthcoming due to their fear of seeming "like a failure").

(Continued)

Table 7.2 (Continued)

Thought Environment: Common Types of Thought Patterns and Suggested Exploration Activities	
Thought Pattern	Basic Activities and Discussions to Illustrate Thought Patterns
	If the child agrees they have excessive negative thinking and wants to address it, the therapist may proceed to invite the child to change their thought environment by activating the opposites of the negative thought patterns. One way to do this is to present the child with another worksheet with space to describe a situation or situations where they predominantly used negative self-talk, and what the "cloudy voice" actually said.[a] Then encourage the child to activate its opposite (the "sunny voice"), and write it down. For example, if the child was extremely upset with themselves for scoring lower than expected on a test where the cloudy voice may have said, "I am never going to get better as this", its opposite voice could say, "I will give it another try".
Inflexible thinking, or only one way of viewing the motives and intents of others, and difficult or problematic situations,[b] expressed as:	
Being critical and/or rude towards others, and controlling in certain situations	Two-part activity: Play dough and wooden block, role play. 1) Use play dough and ask the child to shape it into an object of their choice, e.g. a car or cat. Then give the child a solid object such as a wooden block and ask them to shape it into the same object as they did with the play dough, which is obviously not possible. Follow with a discussion on flexible or "play dough thinking" vs. inflexible or "solid thinking" and how these help or do not help us to view other people and situations in a different way. Being able to view people or situations differently can help us feel regulated and also resolve conflicts and problems easier. Follow with: 2) Asking the child about one or two difficult situations they were in, and whether on reflection they think they were using flexible or inflexible thinking with regards to the people and/or situations. Use simple role play where the therapist and child act out the scenarios, with the child first using solid thinking, and then repeating the role play, this time asking the child to use play dough thinking. Ask the child afterwards to discuss how they felt in each roleplay scenario.
Emotional outbursts	See "concern with justice and fairness" below.
Concern with justice and fairness, expressed as:	
Preoccupation with problems often affecting activity participation, but with associated drive to solve problems	Precede this activity by asking the child's parent or carer to list up to ten current issues and/or situations that the child is overly concerned with and/or experiences as problematic. Three-part activity: Famous problem quote, problem classification, general and personal problem classification.

(Continued)

Copyright material from Mariza Ferreira and Rebecca Howell (2024), *Occupational Therapy for Children with DME or Twice Exceptionality*, Routledge

Table 7.2 (Continued)

Thought Environment: Common Types of Thought Patterns and Suggested Exploration Activities	
Thought Pattern	Basic Activities and Discussions to Illustrate Thought Patterns

	1) When asked how he would order his thoughts if he had one hour to save the world, Albert Einstein said he would spend 55 minutes of the hour thinking about the problem before using the remainder of the time working on solutions. Read the complete quote (found online) and use it to lead on a discussion about defining or classifying problems being a crucial step in solving them, since classifying problems can help with the speed with which they are solved.
	2) Use a problem classification system such as "easy", "hard" and "complex"[c] and write these on three separate cards, i.e. "easy problem", "hard problem" and "complex problem", and stick these on a wall using sticky tack. Then write the definition of each type of problem on separate cards as below:
	   a. Easy – a problem that is simple, well understood, requires little thought, and can be solved easily and/or quickly
	   b. Hard – a problem that is fairly straightforward and has an obvious solution, but which takes longer (or is more difficult) to solve due to emotional-, moral- or value-based reasons
	   c. Complex – a problem that is not well defined and/or takes time and effort to fully understand. It is very important to find a solution in a timely manner before the problem gets worse, but there are no obvious right answers or solutions and therefore it takes a longer time to resolve
	Hide the problem definition cards in a bucket filled with beads, rice etc., taking into account any allergies and sensory sensitivities the child may have. Ask the child to lie prone on a scooter board and scoot forward to collect one card from the bucket, and on the return stick the definition card under the problem type they think it relates to. Repeat with the other two cards. Discuss the pairings as necessary.
	3) Beforehand, write a few everyday situations for each type of problem on separate cards (see below for ideas), as well as the specific problems the child's parent or carer has provided beforehand – ensuring they are adapted to appear generic.
	   a. You forget to set the oven timer and burn the cake you are baking as a result (easy)
	   b. You are playing your favourite online game, but your mother tells you to stop as you need to leave for an appointment (easy)
	   c. You were looking forward to visiting your cousin who lives far away, but he calls to let you know he is too unwell and you have to cancel the visit (hard)
	   d. You have a 2pm appointment with your doctor, but it is now 3pm and you are still waiting. You have to be at your friend's birthday party at 3:30pm. You now feel worried (hard)
	   e. The coronavirus pandemic that started affecting the world in 2020 (complex)
	   f. Large scale floods in areas due to excessive rain (complex)
	Repeat activity (2) for each situation card, being aware that children with DME/2e may not place certain problem situations under the typically expected type of problem. This can be very valuable to promote discussions on how they view and feel about certain problems. Together with the below activity designed to address emotional outbursts, it can help them gain insight into their feelings and reactions to certain problems and whether they feel regulated or "up to the task" of solving the problem and, if not, what they can do about it.

(Continued)

Table 7.2 (Continued)

Thought Environment: Common Types of Thought Patterns and Suggested Exploration Activities	
Thought Pattern	Basic Activities and Discussions to Illustrate Thought Patterns
Emotional outbursts that are out of context to the situation	Three-part activity: problem and feelings balancing metaphor, visually representing the balance, personal application of balancing problem and feelings. (Note, this activity has the most impact when presented after the three-part activity to address 'preoccupation with problems'). (1) Start by stating that just as the scale of justice is about balanced or fair representation of the two sides of a case in court, so our feelings must be balanced with the type of problem in order to help us solve it. (2) Have a homemade hanger and paper cup scale[d] to hand (or make one with the child if they like creating things and/or if time allows) and write "type of problem" on one cup, and "a person's feelings about it" on the other cup. Now use weights and ask the child to add weights to the problem cup to represent an easy problem (will most likely only be a few weights) followed by adding weights to the feelings cup so that it balances out (has to be the same amount of weights). Repeat for a hard problem and then for a complex problem. (3) Now refer to one or more of the child-specific problem situations discussed in the "drive to solve problems three-part activity" and ask the child to represent both the type of problem and their real life feelings about it with the weights. Whether their feelings balance out with the type of problem or not, this can lead to important discussions about whether they feel regulated enough (or "up to the task") to address the problem. If not, the therapist can ask them whether there are any sensory, thought or other strategies they can use to help them feel more regulated in order to more easily address and solve the problem.

[a] Sparks, D. (2019, May 29). Mayo Mindfulness: Overcoming negative self-talk. *Mayo Clinic.* https://newsnetwork.mayoclinic.org/discussion/mayo-mindfulness-overcoming-negative-self-talk/. Adapted.
[b] Cambridge Dictionary. (n.d.) *Inflexible.* In Dictionary.cambridge.org. https://dictionary.cambridge.org/dictionary/english/inflexible. Adapted.
[c] Karle, D. (2019, September 10) Three Types of Problems. *LinkedIn Article* https://www.linkedin.com/pulse/three-types-problems-dave-karle/.
[d] Agrawal, G.K. (2016, May 17) *How to make a balance scale for kids at home.* [Video]. YouTube. https://www.youtube.com/watch?v=7Prz7n8cD9Q.

An example of how to use S-TE-DD-R for negative thought patterns expressed as being self-critical and having inner dialogue or negative self-talk

Although we advise therapists dedicate specific sessions to exploring the unhelpful thought patterns impacting a child with DME/2e, the reality is that therapists can address these subtly from the start of intervention and throughout. Ways to achieve this are through adopting the optimum approach for the child (the 10 Golden Nuggets) and "tapping into" some of the common characteristics of children with HLP the child displays, such as their strong curiosity and having compassion for others. For instance, if the therapist has identified the child has excessive or intense negative thought patterns, such as being overly self-critical and/or having constant negative self-talk to the extent of it affecting their academic performance but also has strong compassion for others, then having a discussion about being

The DME-C Approach's Four Walls 151

your own "best friend" may be suitable at any point in therapy (see Table 7.2 Negative thought patterns). Piquing the child's curiosity by doing the grass head activity a couple of weeks before the session in which the therapist plans to explore self-talk can help to reinforce the concept of the effect self-talk has on the child's life.

With regards to the session in which self-talk is addressed (among other thought patterns), the therapist should provide the child with a written summary of the key elements explored during the session, as well as the self-talk worksheet done in the session. The child should continue to use this in the following weeks for a situation or situations in which they identify using predominantly negative self-talk and what the opposite positive self-talk to that would be. The therapist should also make sure they discuss the homework at the start of the next session with the child. Figure 7.7 shows an example of a session summary sheet. Please note it is an extract only as generally other thought patterns would also have been covered in the session, such as perfectionism and flexible thinking.

Figure 7.7 An extract of a session summary sheet with related occupational therapy homework for thought environment.

An extract of a session summary sheet with related occupational therapy homework
Child: Date of session:
Session number: Venue:
Persons present:

Today we explored:

- Using kind words to encourage a friend going through a difficult situation.
- That we all use self-talk, and that this can be positive or negative. We completed a worksheet to help us understand what this is.
  - Positive self-talk is the sunny (or optimistic) voice in your head that helps you feel "up to the task" – whatever that may be!
  - Negative self-talk is the cloudy (or pessimistic) voice in your head that makes it hard for you to "feel up to the task" – whatever that may be!
- By using a worksheet, we identified a situation or situations in the past where you may have used negative self-talk and what your "cloudy voice" actually said, as well as what the "sunny voice" could have said instead.
- The reason for doing the grass head activity a few weeks ago.

Today we learnt that:

- We can be our "own best friend" by using kind words to encourage ourselves in difficult situations, just like we would a close friend.
- We need to consider the impact of self-talk on how we feel, but that we can change how we feel if needed by:
  - Identifying unhelpful thought patterns, in this case negative thinking and self-talk, and deciding to change our thought environment.
  - Helping the thought patterns that are struggling by activating their opposites, in this case using positive thinking and self-talk.
- The "voice" we listen to the most, will have the biggest impact on our lives.

The OT homework to complete before the next session:
Use the self-talk worksheet we started with in the session, and if you come across situations in the next couple of weeks where you catch yourself using the cloudy voice, activate its opposite and write down what the sunny voice would say instead.

Essential Component 4: Communicate

- Main aim: To help a child with DME/2e find the words to describe their own feelings, experiences and responses to sensory- and thought-based triggers. This promotes self-awareness and relationships with the child's family and significant others

Communicate means to "find or develop a common language" that will help a child with DME/2e and their parents or carers talk about their challenges with regard to their sensory needs, thought life and feelings. It is finding words and terminology they are comfortable with and which they can use in order to describe "where they are at" to each other, the child's teachers and other relevant adults when advocating for themselves/their child.

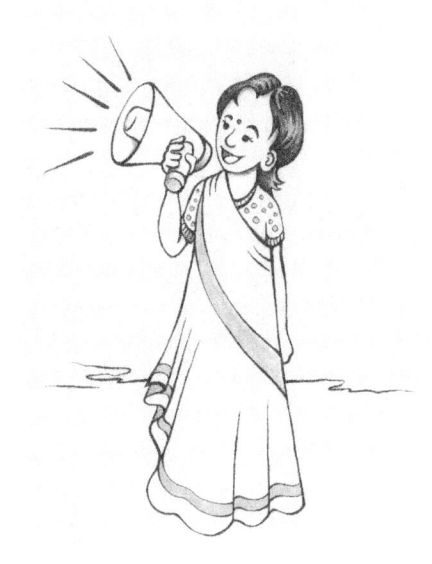

It is not uncommon for children with DME/2e to feel there is "something seriously wrong" with them prior to occupational therapy. They are often aware they are different to their peers, not just cognitively and in how they think about the world, but in how they perceive and react to sensory input. However, they are frequently unable to put adequate words to these differences and feelings. In most cases, children with DME/2e and their parents report a huge sense of relief when they enter the therapy process and learn that what they experience has a "name", can be defined, is also experienced by other children and can be addressed. "Communicate" is highly empowering and therefore an imperative part of the therapy process.

Helping a child with DME/2e "find a language" is a concept that is introduced at the start of therapy and developed throughout its progression to make it more bespoke for the individual child. There are two main ways to achieve this, which are:

1. Using a visual metaphor
2. The therapist modelling how to use "communicate" during sessions

Using a visual metaphor

A visual metaphor is a **visual aid** where a concept is represented by a visual image and/or object to help the child understand it better. For example, a "feelings thermometer" filled with the colours green, blue, yellow, orange and red in ascending order can represent the feelings happy and calm, sad, worried, frustrated and angry.

The ability to self-regulate, and the need for therapy and resources to help children with associated challenges achieve this, have increasingly been in the spotlight over the last few years and we believe this will continue to be the case in future. As a result, there is extensive information and a number of programmes and resources[†] available to help children. Therapists may be aware of well-established and emerging programs by occupational therapists, other professionals and parents such as: The Incredible 5-Point Scale,[6] The Alert Program®,[7] The Zones of Regulation®,[8] Autism Level UP!™ (www.autismlevelup.com), Sensory Ladders (www.sensoryladders.org), Mindfulmazing (www.mindfulmazing.com), Big Life Journal (www.biglifejournal.com) and Mind Ninja (lifelessonsglobal.com/mindninja) to name but a few. Most programs make use of some kind of visual aid, and we also highly value this method to help children "develop a language".

Visual aids can be a combination of colours, pictures of people's faces with a range of emotions, words, and rating scales such as one to five, slow to fast, cold to hot, etc. to help children better identify and understand "where they are at", such as feeling angry, bored or misunderstood in addition to their associated behaviours, such as crying, saying unkind words or breaking furniture.

Choosing which visual aid to use will differ from one therapist to another. When therapists work with children with DME/2e individually in their own clinical settings, they may find they use only one visual aid, they combine visual aids, or they quickly move away from these aids to create a new one in collaboration with the child with DME/2e who has inadvertently made connections between the metaphor/s and one which corresponds more with their particular areas of interest. It is therefore recommended that children are given the opportunity to make their own visual aids in therapy, which they can take home and share with others. This will ultimately promote family relationships and the ability of the child and their parents or carers to advocate for their needs more effectively.

Therapists should also be aware that children with DME/2e may link certain feelings with parts of the visual aids in unexpected ways. For example, they may link feeling intellectually bored with the sensory seeking behaviour of excessive fidgeting, or following five different group conversations in class as helping them feel invigorated and "just right" for learning instead of overwhelmed.

Therapist modelling the use of a "common language"

Therapists can help a child with DME/2e develop a language to describe their feelings and behaviours in everyday situations by modelling how to use words and terminology as they develop throughout the therapy process. For example, a therapist may say to a child with tactile defensiveness (sensory trigger), "You have described that you are always **irritated** and **fighting** with your siblings during car journeys. Could it be that **sitting physically close** to them makes you feel so **uncomfortable** that you just want to **lash out** at them?" Or for a child with a highly developed sense of "right and wrong" who is extremely upset as the rules of a tennis match they played were not consistently applied by the overseeing adult (thought trigger related to external circumstances), the therapist may say, "From what you have described I agree that the **game's rules were not applied correctly**. It is understandable that you were **incredibly upset** and **unable to play your best game** as a result. Can we explore together how to handle similar situations in the future that may be out of your control?"

Through modelling the use of a common language, the therapist is also helping the child with DME/2e and their parents understand that the child's feelings, whether because of sensory- or thought-based triggers, often have a direct connection to their ability to self-regulate and participate appropriately in everyday activities.

It is important the therapist acknowledges all of the child with DME/2e's feelings regardless of the sensory- or thought-based triggers and/or circumstances, as the child needs to understand it is acceptable and human to experience a range of emotions. The therapist and child can then explore whether the child was able to self-regulate appropriately in certain situations and, if not, work together to find suitable sensory- and thought-based (or other) strategies for similar situations in the future.

The 4 Essential Components Working Together

The DME-C therapy approach's four walls, or 4 Essential Components of **D**iarise, **M**anage transitions, change the **E**nvironment and h**E**lp the senses and **C**ommunicate, can only be effective if they are interwoven and working together throughout the therapy process.

Using **Diarise**, children with DME/2e and their parents or carers are able to start identifying and, with time, anticipating the situations and their associated triggers in which children feel dysregulated and not "up to the task", whatever that task may be. **change the Environment and hElp the senses** further assists them to develop increased self-awareness of how their sensory and thought environments affect their feelings and behaviours. **Communicate** helps children find the words to describe these environments, to better express their thoughts and feelings and to advocate for themselves. Children will find the use of schedules (part of **manage transitions**) helpful to anticipate potentially stressful situations, and through the use of **change the Environment and hElp the senses** learn the principles of developing their own effective coping or management strategies to address their individual sensory and thought environments.

Conclusion

Having read Chapter 7, it is our hope therapists will understand the importance of including the 4 Essential Components in their therapy provision for children with DME/2e. It is our aim to encourage therapists that they indeed have the skills to adapt activities to achieve the 4 Essential Components to effectively meet the needs of children with DME/2e. Indeed, when teaching the DME-C therapy approach to occupational therapists in person, they have reported they feel able to immediately include the 4 Essential Components into their therapy provision for children with DME/2e, and/or they are already including these elements but in future they will focus more on tailoring activities. We trust, having provided example activities throughout Chapter 7 of how to do this, we have inspired therapists to do the same.

In the next chapter, we will discuss the parts of everyday OT work that are not the therapy itself and how to include provision for DME/2e in this. We will look at what the most important factors of the occupational therapy process are for therapists to consider when assessing and treating a child with DME/2e, including report writing following assessment and highlighting the child's needs – both with regards to their high learning potential (or giftedness), their special educational need or disability (or learning difference), goal setting, re-evaluation and further referral if needed.

Notes

* Covertly, in this context, means using the strategies in sessions without calling the child's attention directly to them but not deliberately attempting to hide/obfuscate them.
† Note: The authors have listed some self-regulation programmes for information purposes only, and do not endorse or dissuade therapists from any one programme. Using and adapting materials and/or terminology from therapeutic programmes is acceptable in the context of personal use by the therapist in their own clinical setting and one-to-one work with children.

References

1. Cambridge dictionary. (n.d.) Transition. *In Dictionary.Cambridge.org*. Retrieved on February 1, 2023, from https://dictionary.cambridge.org/dictionary/english/transition.
2. PDA Society (n.d.) What is demand avoidance? https://www.pdasociety.org.uk/what-is-pda-menu/what-is-demand-avoidance/.
3. Millard, E. (2021, March 30) Prolonged Focus on Negative Moments may Impact Mental Health. *Very Well Mind*. https://www.verywellmind.com/focus-on-negative-moments-impacts-mental-health-5119174.
4. Cuncic, A. (2021, June 22) Amygdala Hijack and the Fight or Flight Response. *Very Well Mind*. https://www.verywellmind.com/what-happens-during-an-amygdala-hijack-4165944.
5. Stierwalt, S. (2020, June 29) Why do smells trigger memories? Scientific American. https://www.scientificamerican.com/article/why-do-smells-trigger-memories1/.
6. Buron, K. D. & Curtis, M. (2003) The Incredible Five Point Scale. AAPC Publishing.
7. Williams, M.S., & Shellenberger, S. (1996). How Does Your Engine Run?: A leader's guide to the Alert Program® for self-regulation. Albuquerque, NM: TherapyWorks, Inc.
8. Kuypers, L. (2011) The Zones of Regulation™: A curriculum designed to foster self-regulation and emotional control. Think Social Publishing.

Chapter eight
Making DME/2e Part of Everyday Occupational Therapy Work

Introduction

As with any occupational therapy, it is important to follow the occupational therapy process when working with children with DME/2e. In a nutshell, the process involves referral ⇒ screening ⇒ evaluation or assessment ⇒ goal setting ⇒ intervention planning and implementation ⇒ re-evaluation ⇒ discharge from therapy, continuing with therapy and/or further referral.

In this chapter, we will briefly discuss the most important factors of the occupational therapy process to consider when assessing and treating a child with DME/2e, including report writing following assessment to highlight the child's needs – both with regards to their high learning potential (or giftedness) and their special educational need or disability (or learning difference), goal setting, re-evaluation and further referral if needed.

Evaluation or Assessment

Once a therapist agrees to work with a child, we would suggest a thorough assessment is done of the child's occupational performance areas and the strengths and challenges that may be affecting their activity participation. We appreciate it may not always be possible to do full assessments and/or write full reports due to departmental policies, constraints on funding and resources or another reason. However, we do advise that as comprehensive an assessment as possible is carried out, as this will provide a holistic view of the child and will therefore inform therapy as best as possible.

Prior to the actual assessment session or sessions with a child, the therapist can gather information about the child by way of interviews with, in addition to informal and formal questionnaires completed by, the child's parents, carers or teachers and other relevant reports by other occupational therapists, educational psychologists, psychiatrists and assessors from organisations such as Mensa or Potential Plus UK that have been made available.

When directly assessing a child, we suggest the therapist uses a combination of informal discussions and clinical observations during functional activities and standardised tests to determine the child's activity participation challenges and any related sensory, motor- and self-regulation difficulties. Interpretation and analysis of these will lead to the setting of

DOI: 10.4324/9781003334033-8

Making DME/2e Part of Everyday OT Work 157

therapy goals, where therapists can use standardised goal setting and outcome measures, or functional goals, but still with measurable outcomes.

Report Writing

Many of the occupational therapists who we have trained in person in the DME-C approach have reported they have concerns and/or are unsure how to refer to a child as having, or possibly having, DME/2e in reports and other formal documentation they may produce. We have discussed these concerns and our thoughts about them in the introduction to Chapter 6 and in light of this, we want to encourage therapists to:

- Remember that DME/2e is a term to describe and better understand a child's profile. It is not a diagnosis or condition
- Include a definition of DME/2e in their formal documentation such as reports and letters
- Gather as much evidence as possible regarding a child's profile: their characteristics, strengths and challenges. When a child's cognitive ability has already been confirmed through formal testing or high learning potential is suspected, and the therapist has identified specific challenges through assessment, then the therapist can highlight the term or profile of DME/2e as applicable or possibly applicable to the child. It is essential that both a child's high learning potential and their identified difficulties are recognised and addressed by professionals and educators to enable the child to have the right combination of challenge and support to help them thrive. Below are some extracts from the conclusion sections of reports for children with DME/2e, by way of example.

Assessment Conclusion: Three extracts

Cara

Confirmed as having high learning potential before the occupational therapy assessment.

Cara has high learning potential (see report by … dated xxx). The occupational therapy assessment also confirms that she has definite sensory processing differences, with a mixed profile of sensitivity to auditory and tactile sensory stimulation from the environment, and low registration with regards to visual sensory input from the environment more or much more than others her age. This is affecting her ability to appropriately participate in home and school life. In particular, it affects her ability to **self-regulate**, i.e. to focus and concentrate on relevant tasks, and have emotionally appropriate responses as expected for her age, such as reacting aggressively when accidently touched by one of her peers.

In addition to Cara's sensory processing differences, the assessment process has highlighted she may have an inherent motor coordination difficulty with her motor skills being in line with the features of *development coordination disorder as tested on the Movement ABC-2 standardised test.

Cara fits the profile of having dual or multiple exceptionality (DME), also known as twice exceptionality (2e); she is cognitively more able or has high learning potential (HLP) and also has special educational needs or disabilities – in this case, sensory processing differences combined with motor coordination difficulties. Children with DME/2e are often acutely aware that they struggle to participate in certain tasks, but they are unable to pinpoint the sensory- and motor-based underlying reasons. This can lead to feelings of frustration and low self-esteem affecting their behaviour.

Furthermore, there are other factors that can impact a child with DME/2e's self-esteem and behaviour, including in a social context, and these factors or characteristics are commonly recognised amongst children with HLP. Most noticeably, Cara displays strong perfectionistic traits and asynchronous development with a disparity between her cognitive abilities and social skills, the latter of which lags behind that of her peers. It is thought these factors contribute to her frequent and extreme emotional outbursts...

*Please note that a formal diagnosis of DCD can only be made by a consultant paediatrician whose opinion should be sought as deemed fit.

Otto

High learning potential suspected by parents prior to occupational therapy assessment.

The occupational therapist did not carry out any cognitive assessments with Otto, and his parents reported they had not yet taken him for formal testing. However, he interacted very well with the occupational therapist during the assessment, displaying an extensive and advanced vocabulary as well as significant insight into world issues such as the war in Ukraine, which is beyond the expectation for his age. The occupational therapist would therefore recommend that Otto is tested to determine his cognitive abilities so suitable accommodations can be made to support his learning needs.

Otto has sensory processing differences, and although he achieved an overall standard score of four and percentile rank of 2% on the MABC-2 standardised test, which places his overall motor coordination abilities in the "significant movement difficulty" range, his observed performance of everyday motor skills tasks are as expected for his age and his parents report no concerns in this regard. The occupational therapist suggests there are some non-motor factors that have affected his performance in the various MABC-2 subtasks, such as his observed difficulty focussing during the assessment. Further investigation by a child psychiatrist or other suitable professional may be prudent to rule out or confirm whether he has an attention disorder.

Otto fits the profile of having dual or multiple exceptionality (DME) or twice exceptionality (2e)... [Text continues as in the example above.]

There are factors commonly recognised amongst children with HLP that can impact on their self-esteem and behaviour which apply to Otto. In particular, Otto currently has a fixed mind-set and can be described as having perfectionist tendencies. He sets high expectations for himself, and when he is not able to meet those expectations, it leads to disappointment, frustration and anger. One example of this seen within the assessment was that Otto seemed to "freeze" when asked to write on a topic of his choice, for which he needed guidance as well as support to become calm. After the assessment Otto told the occupational therapist that part of the reason for him freezing was that he was afraid to "make the wrong choice" about which topic to choose.

The occupational therapist is of the opinion that Otto will be able to develop better self-regulation techniques and strategies, but that all adults and professionals working with him need to be aware of his specific needs in order to work together to allow the best chance of success.

Lachelle

Confirmed as having high learning potential before the occupational therapy assessment.

Lachelle has high learning potential (see report by … dated xxx). The occupational therapy assessment confirms she has no movement difficulties, although she has definite sensory processing differences that are affecting her ability to appropriately concentrate in class. In particular, Lachelle has a mixed profile of sensitivity to auditory and visual sensory stimulation from the environment and a need for significantly more movement (vestibular input) than her peers. This results in her frequently approaching her teacher to clarify work for which she already knows the answers.

Lachelle has excellent social skills and reported she has a wide group of friends at school. She also has an awareness of her sensory needs being different from her peers, and will ask her teacher at various times throughout the day whether she may run up and down the stairs outside of her classroom to help her "recalibrate". This awareness is a good foundation to build on to help her further understand and manage her needs as appropriate in various situations.

Lachelle fits the profile of having DME… [Text continues as in example above.]

Goal Setting

As discussed throughout this book, goal setting needs to be done together with the child and their family to ensure they are invested in the therapy process. In most cases, goal setting is aligned between the therapist, child and parent, but in some cases, the child may choose to address goals that the parent and/or therapist may not view as a high priority initially. However, the child's views should be respected, and therapy should be directed accordingly. For example, the parent and therapist may view addressing a child's sensory and thought environments as essential, but the child may want to address his handwriting difficulties first.

For cases in which the focus of therapy includes addressing the child's sensory and thought environments, we suggest an overall therapy goal with shorter term goals for individual sessions, implemented through the DME-C approach. Below we have provided some examples by way of explanation.

Overall therapy goal

For (child name) to develop increased self-awareness of how their sensory experiences and thought processes impact their feelings and behaviours (modulation, self-regulation and activity participation). Furthermore, for (child name) to learn the underlying concepts and principles of developing effective coping strategies for related challenges.

Shorter term goals

Set with the understanding that therapy sessions are lengthened (double sessions).

Sessions 1 and 2
For (child name) to:

- Learn terminology and start developing a language to describe their feelings
- Improve their understanding that their sensory experiences and thought patterns can influence their feelings and/or behaviours
- Become aware that sensory and thought based strategies can help change how they feel

Sessions 3 and 4
For (child name) to:

- Experience and/or explore each type of sensory stimulation with regards to the vestibular, proprioceptive and tactile sensory systems
- Increase their awareness of sensory inputs they dislike and prefer, the latter of which acts as a base on which to develop bespoke and effective coping strategies to help with self-regulation

Sessions 5 and 6
For (child name) to:

- Experience and/or explore each type of sensory stimulation with regards to the oral, visual and auditory sensory systems
- Increase their awareness of sensory inputs they dislike and prefer, the latter of which can act as a base on which to develop bespoke and effective coping strategies to help with self-regulation

Sessions 7 and 8

For (child name) to:

- Explore the use of daily and/or weekly schedules to reduce anxiety related to transitions
- Explore the negative impact of preoccupation with problems on activity participation, and discover how the classification of problems can assist with the speed of solving them
- Explore the necessary balance between the types of problems and a person's feelings about it. Also, to gain insight into their own feelings and reactions to certain problems, whether they feel regulated or "up to the task" of solving them, and if not, what strategies they can implement to help them feel more regulated in order to solve the problems

Sessions 9 and 10

For (child name) to:

- Explore the impact of perfectionism and an associated fear of failure on self-regulation and activity participation
- Explore the impact of positive and negative thinking patterns with associated self-talk on emotions, self-regulation and activity participation
- Explore the impact of flexible and inflexible thinking patterns on emotions, self-regulation, the ability to socialise with others and deal with difficult situations
- Review what they have learnt and gained from therapy and determine further steps

Re-evaluation

In reality, the evaluation of the effectiveness of therapy and whether the overall and shorter term goals are being reached is done throughout the therapy process. As equal partners in the therapy process, children with DME/2e and their parents will most likely provide regular feedback on how they are experiencing therapy, what they feel they are gaining from it, what they think could be done differently and what they would like to add. We encourage therapists to be open to feedback and adjust therapy as needed to ensure the child gains the most from the process. It is also valuable to get more formal feedback at the end of therapy from parents and children, if they choose to give it, which will help therapists to constantly evolve and improve on their therapy provision for children with DME/2e.

Formal feedback from a fourteen-year-old child with DME/2e

The techniques the therapist showed me were useful and easy to do and were things I had not thought of before. She explained things well and repeated things when I needed her to and didn't get impatient. The therapy room was a good open safe space to learn. The best bit was the scooter board! The only thing I would change was maybe some of the craft stuff, as it was aimed at children younger than myself. Did the sessions help me? YES!

We would also advise offering a follow-up session between one and six months after the end of therapy with the child and their parents or carers, either in person or online. This is to determine how they have been managing to deal with their sensory and thought environments in light of what they have learnt in therapy, and whether they feel they need further support from the therapist. In our experience, children with DME/2e generally take the lead with whether and when they would like to have a follow up session and will ask their parents to get in touch with the therapist as needed.

Further Referral

When a therapist starts working with a child with DME/2e, the child may already be working with another professional such as a child psychologist or speech and language therapist. In most cases, occupational therapy can be provided alongside other input if it has been determined with the child and their parents or carers that the child would not feel "overloaded" by this. We would recommend the occupational therapist and other professional liaise during this time to ensure their input is complementary.

The need for input from another professional or organisation, other than an occupational therapist, may only have been identified during the occupational therapy assessment. The same reasoning as above should be followed to determine whether such input should be provided simultaneously, or after, occupational therapy.

There are some rare occasions when occupational therapists may decide it would be in the child's best interest to discontinue therapy even if the therapy program has not yet been completed. For example, as the therapist and child work together, it may become apparent that the child is not truly motivated to work on the goals agreed upon following the assessment. As we work with the belief that children are equal partners in the therapy process, and that successful therapy outcomes rely heavily on children being motivated to fully participate, we suggest having an open, direct and non judgemental discussion with the child about discontinuing therapy. The child should be assured that he can request to restart with occupational therapy at any point in the future.

Another example where it may be best to discontinue therapy is when a child who has engaged in sessions suddenly displays unexpected and unanticipated, significant negative and emotionally explosive behaviours during a session, resulting in them withdrawing from the session and being unable to re-engage successfully in that or further sessions despite the therapist, child and parent talking through the incident at a time when the child has calmed down. This behaviour may have suspected roots in severe depression and/or anxiety, post-traumatic stress disorder and attachment difficulties or other yet unidentified mental health or psychological difficulties, which the DME-C approach is not designed to address. At such times an urgent referral to the child's doctor, paediatrician, psychologist or other appropriate child mental health professional should be made.

Making DME/2e Part of Everyday OT Work 163

There are also a number of other professionals and organisations occupational therapists should be aware of in order to refer children and their families as needed. This will reassure therapists that they are not the only professionals who can help children with HLP and DME/2e, especially when the help needed clearly falls outside the remit or scope of occupational therapy. We have listed some of these professionals and organisations in Chapter 10, but please be aware we do not personally endorse them and children with DME/2e and their families will need to determine for themselves whether the services on offer are suitable for their individual needs.

Conclusion

In Chapter 8, we have highlighted the most important parts of the occupational therapy process that we believe therapists may initially have difficulty with when they start working with children with DME/2e. Even though taking this step may seem daunting at first, we want to encourage therapists to take on the challenge of working with children with DME/2e as occupational therapy is, in our opinion, the vital link for helping them. In Chapter 9, we will provide ten case studies to further help therapists in their understanding of how to use the DME-C approach to guide their work.

Chapter nine
Case Studies

Introduction

In this chapter, we share ten case studies of children who have DME/2e where the challenges most of them wanted to work on first related to sensory processing differences and/or unhelpful thought patterns that impacted their ability to appropriately self-regulate. The sensory processing differences and thought patterns had been identified as part of the occupational therapy assessment. Unhelpful/negative thought patterns such as these are often related to high learning potential. With all these case studies, the therapists used the Golden Nuggets they felt were most needed for each child in the method of providing therapy, and they considered the 4 Essential Components for therapy. The case studies are structured by:

- Providing background information
- Highlighting the main occupational therapy assessment findings
- Explaining how therapy was provided
- Ending with the outcome of therapy and direct parent and/or child feedback or summaries of their feedback

We are aware that with most of these case studies, the child's parent and/or carer attended therapy sessions and were highly engaged in the therapy process to help their children. The reason for our choices is because these case studies most accurately reflect the use of the DME-C therapy approach, and therefore aid readers' understanding of how the 10 Golden Nuggets and 4 Essential Components could be used in therapy. However, there will undoubtedly be times when it will not be possible for parents and/or carers to attend therapy sessions. During these times therapists need to use alternative ways to keep parents and carers informed and involved with therapy. We encourage therapists to refer back to Chapter 6, "Golden Nugget 1: Purposefully empower parents/carers alongside children", where we discussed some ideas on how to achieve this.

Prior to reading the case studies, we encourage therapists to have a pen and paper ready, and to also print off the full summary of the DME-C therapy approach found in Figure 9.1. With each case study, therapists should first read the background information and main occupational therapy assessment findings and then, using Figure 9.1 as a guide, consider and write down how they would approach each case. Therapists should then continue to read the rest of the case study to try and identify the combination of Golden Nuggets used, as well as how the therapists achieved the Essential Components. To simplify this, therapists may want to add the Golden Nugget numbers one to ten, and Essential Component

DOI: 10.4324/9781003334033-9

	The DME-C therapy approach: 10 Golden Nuggets & 4 Essential Components Summary
	(illustration of a brick house with blocks labelled M, E, D, C and a figure laying bricks)
	10 Golden Nuggets
1	Purposefully empower parents/carers alongside children
2	Lengthen the sessions
3	Set clear & healthy boundaries from the start
4	Use direct language
5	Monitor your responses
6	Do not repeat previously learned information
7	To make sessions engaging: Include practical and cipher activities
8	To make sessions engaging: Design unexpected or delayed outcomes
9	Find the WOW and Super WOW Factors
10	Foster a growth mindset

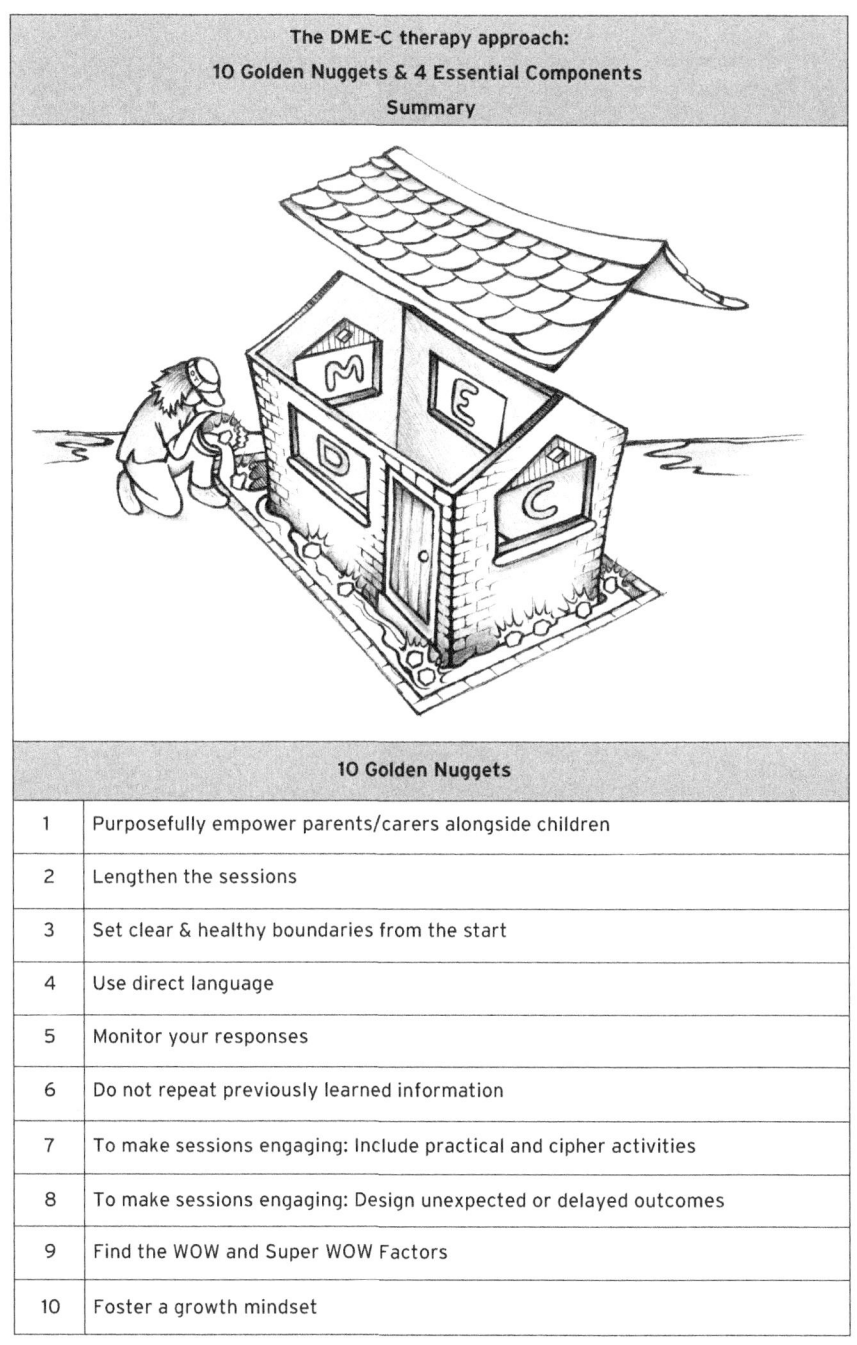

Figure 9.1 The DME-C therapy approach: 10 Golden Nuggets and 4 Essential Components summary. M Ferreira, R Howell.

Copyright material from Mariza Ferreira and Rebecca Howell (2024),
Occupational Therapy for Children with DME or Twice Exceptionality, Routledge

		4 Essential Components
D	**Diarise**	
	• Keep a diary or journal for 3 to 4 days	
M	**Manage transitions**	
	• Use strategies covertly during therapy sessions 　○ Use visual schedules to demonstrate session progression 　○ Discuss the next activity before the current one is finished • Purposefully explore management strategies in sessions 　○ Devise daily or weekly schedules 　○ Explore specific transition activities	
E	**change the Environment and hElp the senses**	
	• Follow the "**S-TE-DD-R**" (or *steadier)* guidelines of: 　○ **Subdivide** ⇒ **Teach & Experience /Explore** ⇒ **Discuss & Discover** ⇒ **Remember** • For the sensory environment, with Discuss & Discover: 　○ **Change** the physical environment with its sensory elements. 　○ **Help** the sensory system that is "struggling" by using the same sensory system (or sense) but in a different way. 　○ **Help** the sensory system that is "struggling" by activating another sensory system (or sense). • For the thought environment, with Discuss & Discover: 　○ **Change** the unhelpful thought patterns in the thought environment. 　○ **Help** the thought patterns that are "struggling" by activating their opposites.	
C	**Communicate**	
	• Use a visual metaphor or visual aid • Model the use of a "common language"	

letters D, M, E and C, next to the relevant text. This will help therapists build on their knowledge and understanding of how to help children with DME/2e. It has been our experience, when presenting our course on occupational therapy for children with HLP and DME/2e in person to occupational therapists, that therapists ask insightful questions, have further suggestions to enhance therapy and are able to immediately think of ways they can start incorporating the DME-C approach into their therapy provision for children with DME/2e.

CASE STUDY 1: SALLY

Background

Sally was an eight-year-old girl (Year 3 in England and Wales) with confirmed high learning potential. She was very creative and artistic, had a love for acting and also had leadership qualities with a strong sense of right and wrong or "how things should be done". Sally was referred to occupational therapy by her parents, with their main concerns being that she was struggling with her sensory issues and managing her emotions. Sally's parents reported that at school she particularly struggled with the unstructured and enclosed nature of the breakfast club she attended, and that she often reported getting headaches when in this environment. Furthermore, her parents reported she would change from being completely calm to exceptionally angry and upset in a matter of seconds, displaying destructive and harmful behaviours towards herself, her two younger siblings and property. During these times, she also sometimes said that she wanted to end her life as she saw this as the only way to end her strong negative emotions. After Sally had calmed down, she would be genuinely upset and embarrassed about her behaviour, with extensive negative self-talk where she berated and blamed herself, which in turn influenced her self-esteem.

Prior to occupational therapy Sally's parents had been working closely with her school to try and help her recognise the triggers for her behaviour and use de-escalation strategies, but they reported it had mixed success. The strategies they were already using included distraction, listening to audio books, completing a creative task, deep breathing, counting and going outside for some fresh air.

Sally's parents wanted her to get help before things got worse. They were struggling to know how best to support her beyond what they were already doing and also wanted to know what further advice they could give to her school. After reading up extensively on what options were available to support Sally, they decided on occupational therapy due to its holistic, practical and targeted approach.

Main occupational therapy assessment findings

The occupational therapist carried out a full assessment with the main findings being that Sally had good motor skills, but she was seeking out significantly more movement than her peers. This was sometimes problematic, e.g. when her teacher wanted her

168 *Case Studies*

to sit down for a lesson but she felt she needed to stand or move around. Sally was particularly sensitive to noisy environments, which in the absence of a medical reason, was thought to be contributing to the headaches she was getting at the breakfast club. She also had perfectionistic tendencies and set high standards for herself and possibly others such as her siblings, but she did not yet have the emotional maturity to cope if her expectations were not met.

Sally was forthcoming from the start of her interaction with the occupational therapist. She acknowledged she was struggling to make sense of and deal with her strong negative emotions and was therefore highly motivated to work with the therapist.

Stop! Consider and write down how you would approach working with Sally, keeping the 10 Golden Nuggets and 4 Essential Components in mind.

Therapy provision and outcome

The therapist worked with Sally over five double sessions, each lasting one-and-a-half hours. Sally's parents took turns attending sessions and would afterwards discuss the sessions with each other. Sally particularly enjoyed the practical element of sessions, so the therapist ensured to include as many practical activities as possible. For example, in the first double session, Sally made her own visual aid, which in her case was to combine the speedometer from The Alert Program® [1] with the colours from The Zones of Regulation® [2]. However, she personalised it further by drawing and individually colouring triangle-shaped characters with different facial expressions, which she glued to the visual aid. In another session, during which the therapist explored the necessary balance between the types of problems and a person's feelings about it, the therapist asked Sally to make a basic hanger and paper cup scale in the session instead of presenting her with a pre-made one.

By keeping a diary (or journal) over the course of three non-consecutive days, the therapist and Sally were able to determine that one main sensory-based trigger responsible for some of her emotional outbursts (or dysregulated state) was that she was always unable to cope with noisy car journeys with her siblings. Also, the main thought-based triggers responsible for some of Sally's outbursts were that she had inflexible thinking patterns about the motives of her younger brother and sister when they played and spent time together. She also became upset when others, e.g. either a classmate she had to work with on a project in school or her sister who tried to imitate her singing, did it "wrong".

Sally and her parents started to develop their own language or vocabulary to describe their feelings, and the therapist followed suit by using the same vocabulary and terms in sessions. She also encouraged them to share this with Sally's SENDCo (special educational needs and disabilities coordinator) and teacher. As therapy progressed, Sally learnt more about various sensory stimuli and thought patterns and how they impacted on the way she felt and behaved. Sally quickly caught onto the principles of developing effective coping strategies for her specific challenges, and turned up to one therapy session reporting that she had made a "sensory box" which included stress balls and ear defenders to use during car journeys. The therapist and Sally also discussed which strategies could help in school during the breakfast club, and Sally's parents agreed to speak to her SENDCo about it.

During sessions, or when discussing situations at home during which Sally became instantly angry, the therapist would in a calm and non-judgemental way describe or point out her unhealthy or inappropriate behaviour. Sally found learning about different types of self-talk insightful although challenging, and of her own accord created and drew a character to represent her negative thought patterns or "voice". She later also created and drew a character to represent her positive thought patterns or "voice", which reminded her to remain "calm and collected"; this was self-talk that she had already adopted prior to occupational therapy but which she now related to her positive voice character.

Sally also eagerly participated in role play in which she first had to use her inflexible or solid thinking patterns followed by using her flexible or play dough thinking patterns. This was for specific situations such as when she played badminton with her brother and how he behaved when he won, or when Sally's sister wanted to use her colouring pens instead of her own. When she had the thoughts "my brother is being mean" or "my sister wants to annoy me" in her head during role play, she reported feeling angry; but when she had the thoughts "my brother is just glad he won" and "my sister looks up to me and that is why she wants to use my pens" in her head, she reported that it made her feel calm and more regulated.

During the last double session, Sally brought along pictures of ten mindfulness strategies that she had learnt about in school, and she and the therapist discussed the ones that she preferred to help her feel more regulated, and whether these strategies were sensory- or thought-based. Discussing her emotional outbursts in particular, Sally was able to identify the warning signs, which were that she started avoiding eye contact with others, made grunting noises, felt her face getting warm and felt restless with an increased need to move. Sally agreed to work with her parents to agree on a word/signal that she could use at such times so that she could quickly remove herself to a safe space where she could use some of her various strategies to feel calmer. Sally was keen to have a follow up session with the therapist after about three to four months, and also agreed to complete a home program during this time.

In the meantime, the therapist had a meeting with Sally's SENDCo in which she discussed her occupational therapy and how this complemented what the school had been doing to help Sally. The therapist and Sally's parents stayed in contact, and Sally had a further two sessions, each lasting 45 minutes and being four months apart. During these sessions

Sally reported she was doing much better with managing her sensory needs and unhelpful thought patterns, mentioned still feeling annoyed when her teacher asked her to sit down for lessons (although she understood it) as she felt she wanted to move, and her siblings doing things "wrong". Together with the therapist, Sally explored further ways to address these challenges, such as "finding a way to be seated and still move" like sitting on an inflatable cushion in class, and doing some more role play where she practised using her play dough thinking. The therapist also did the "paper plate painting with salad spinner" activity with Sally, which created an "aha moment" for her with regards to the idea that other people may do things differently to her but they were not necessarily wrong.

Sally and her parents provided feedback to the therapist throughout the whole therapy process. When providing formal feedback at the end of therapy, they stated they felt the process had fully met their goals and they were satisfied with the outcome of therapy. Among their many comments, Sally's parents reported that the sessions were "life-saving", "personalised and child-led... not a one-size fits all... specific to her needs" and a space where she "felt safe to explore her complex emotions – and this was in no small part down to the relationship the therapist built with her". Sally herself made a card for the therapist with a picture on the front, and the words, "Thank you for helping me. I will miss you loads. I hope you enjoy this card. I have left it blank so you can colour it in. Lots of love from Sally". In her brilliance, Sally had left the therapy process with homework not for herself, but for the therapist!

CASE STUDY 2: MAX

Background

Max was fifteen years old, an only child, living with his parents and home educated since the age of nine, which the family reported worked really well for him. Max's mother was of the opinion that he had high learning potential as he exhibited many traits of giftedness although he had not been formally tested. Max enjoyed his own company, had a variety of interests especially history and nature and reported that he never got bored. Max's mother sought occupational therapy at Max's request, as he had always struggled with sensitivity towards noise. He already had some strategies to deal with his auditory sensitivities, such as always wearing ear defenders when he went to the cinema or theatre, but at other times he would avoid places where there might be loud noises. He wanted to have more strategies so that he could feel confident in noisy environments. His mother also reported that while still in formal schooling his teacher thought he might have dyslexia, he had a very poor short term memory, described himself as generally "very clumsy", and he avoided writing at all cost, doing all of his homeschooling work on the computer. His mother therefore requested a full assessment to determine if he needed help in any other occupational therapy related areas.

Main occupational therapy assessment findings

In addition to Max's auditory sensitivities, the assessment highlighted that he had sensitivities towards visual and tactile input from the environment; he struggled to find objects in competing backgrounds, and he became distressed when standing too close to others. Furthermore, the therapist suggested Max had a retained Moro reflex, as he had excessive startle responses to unexpected noises from the environment. It was thought that all of these factors were contributing to Max avoiding noisy and busy places. With regards to Max's motor skills, he fit the profile of having developmental coordination disorder, the effects of which were most noticeable in his writing (or refusal to do so), and quality of performance of everyday motor tasks including struggling to eat with a knife and fork and often bumping into objects.

Stop! Consider and write down how you would approach working with Max, keeping the 10 Golden Nuggets and 4 Essential Components in mind.

Therapy provision and outcome

The therapist discussed the assessment findings with Max and his mother, and although he reported some relief at having an explanation for his motor skills challenges, his main priority remained to develop better strategies to deal with his auditory sensitivities. The therapist did not identify any particular harmful thought patterns impacting on Max's activity participation, but he opted to still investigate thought-based coping principles alongside sensory-based principles as he was keen to expand his coping strategies in general. Max then attended five double therapy sessions, each lasting one-and-a-half hours, with his mother present for all of the sessions. Max engaged well with all of the activities in sessions, but he was generally quiet, and it was initially difficult for the therapist to gauge whether he found the sessions valuable. Instead, his mother would provide written feedback via email following each double session. Also, even though Max grasped the concepts in therapy very quickly, the therapist had to repeat explanations within sessions to accommodate for his poor short term memory.

An initial "win" for Max was that he and his parents were able to start developing a language to describe his feelings in response to his sensory environment. However, as therapy progressed, it became apparent that Max felt he could not speak up or say when he did not like something or when he felt uncomfortable. For example, during the session in which the therapist helped Max to explore the tactile sensory system, he instantly looked worried when the therapist asked him to wrap himself in his favourite blanket that he had taken along to the session, and he placed it over his head instead. He later told his mother he thought the therapist was going to touch/help him wrap the blanket around himself, and as he did not want to be touched, he "hid" under the blanket without thinking. In sessions following this incident, the therapist started discussing with Max the need to advocate for himself and speak up whenever he felt uncomfortable, whether the reason was related to his sensory environment or something else. The therapist also made a point of encouraging Max to voice his thoughts whenever he appeared uncomfortable in sessions.

Max did not do much of the occupational therapy homework as it was based around writing, although he was given the option to have his mother scribe for him or use his computer. However, he discussed sessions and how he could implement what he was learning, at length with his mother. He also consistently did some basic Moro reflex integration exercises at home with the agreement that he might need to see a reflex integration specialist if his severe startle reflex to unexpected noises continued.

During the time Max attended occupational therapy, his mother reported two specific situations where she felt occupational therapy was starting to make a difference. The first was that Max and his mother attended the theatre and his mother reported that

> for the first time he did not take his ear defenders, although he did sit with his fingers in his ears for some of the time and said that he would probably take them along next time. But, there was no sense of panic like previously if the ear defenders had been forgotten; more a calm assessment of the situation.

Another situation was when Max went to the dentist and whilst he was in the dentist chair, the fire alarm went off unexpectedly. His mother reported,

> Amazingly, Max hardly reacted… I still cannot believe it. The dental nurse said it was just a practice, and he calmly stayed in the chair until the alarm had finished, then carried on chatting. This is a boy who, when he was at school, had to be taken out before practice alarms because if not, it would leave him jumpy for weeks whenever he heard a slight noise. I asked him later if he felt startled inside but just managed to react in a calmer way when at the dentist, but he said he did not feel anything!

At the end of therapy, Max opted to give formal feedback to the therapist and was quite eloquent in his responses which were overall positive and showed how far he had improved with "finding his voice". He later asked for follow up sessions to address some of his motor skills challenges, but this was not possible at the time due to the Covid 19 pandemic and lockdowns that followed.

CASE STUDY 3: AMAL

Background

Amal was a seven-year-old girl (Year 3 in England and Wales) and had been assessed as having a very high IQ. She was interested in everything, loved reading – both fiction and non-fiction books, especially finding out facts about things, enjoyed horse riding, painting and completing complicated puzzles. Amal's parents described her as "trying hard, and wanting to be liked". They requested occupational therapy because they were very concerned that she often had emotional outbursts they felt negatively impacted on her behaviour and her ability to form meaningful friendships with her peers. Amal's parents hoped occupational therapy could help her develop management strategies for whatever was causing her emotional outbursts so she would cope better at home and school.

Main occupational therapy assessment findings

Amal was shy and timid at the start of the assessment and avoided eye contact with the therapist, but as the assessment progressed she relaxed, became more talkative and made more eye contact. The assessment process confirmed Amal had sensory processing differences that were contributing to her observed frequent behaviours of appearing stubborn, having emotional outbursts and interacting with tasks less than her peers. She was extremely sensitive to being touched and frequently became anxious when standing too close to others, flinching, recoiling or responding aggressively when accidentally touched. Amal was sensitive to loud and noisy environments and struggled to concentrate with background noise. Furthermore, she did not seem to register visual information from her environment in a timely manner and often missed written instructions or physical demonstrations by her teacher.

In addition to the above, Amal displayed many of the characteristics of children with high learning potential, which also negatively contributed to her behaviours. She was perfectionistic which typically presented as her being afraid of making mistakes and being unable to halt activities midway; both scenarios often resulted in intense emotional outbursts in class and among her peers. The therapist hypothesised that the disparity (or asynchronous development) between her advanced cognitive abilities and delayed emotional and social skills development further caused her internal confusion which contributed to her shyness and timidness.

Stop! Consider and write down how you would approach working with Amal, keeping the 10 Golden Nuggets and 4 Essential Components in mind.

Therapy provision and outcome

Amal attended five double therapy sessions, each of one-and-a-half hours, with her mother present for all sessions. She was very quick to catch onto the concepts being taught about her sensory environment and diligently did her homework each week to explore sensory-based activities that could help change her regulation state if needed. Amal started to understand she was sensitive to tactile and auditory stimulation more than others and that she sometimes missed visual cues, but she could change her physical environment to help herself, such as standing at the back of the line in class, asking the teacher whether she could wear ear plugs to do her work once instructions had been given or using highlighter pens to highlight important pieces of text when working.

Amal also explored how to use her senses in a different way to help her regulate. She realised when she was able to control tactile input, she could benefit from a range of hand-based tactile inputs. She regularly added activities to her list of strategies such as pushing and rubbing her hands together or finding "squishies", such as making and playing with slime (a mixture of household items that come together to create a polymer substance which acts like both a solid and a liquid, depending on how you play with it, and which has become a very popular activity with children in recent years) and having stress balls to hand. She identified she liked music that built up to a crescendo, regardless of its volume or beat, and created her own playlist that she listened to at night before going to bed. With regards to visual input to help her regulate, Amal started grasping that deep colours helped her feel calm and regulated, so she and her mother discussed making a booklet of felt colours of her choice which she could keep to hand and look at if needed. Amal liked the idea of deep breathing as a way to feel calm and created her own "triangle of deep breathing" to help her remember to breathe in deeply through her nose, hold her breath for a few seconds and then breathe out slowly through her mouth.

Amal benefitted from having a visual schedule of the planned session activities and regularly referred to it as sessions progressed. However, on one occasion the therapist realised that there was not going to be enough time to address all the planned activities in the session and that they had to be carried over to the following one. The therapist prepared Amal for this change in schedule by giving her ample warning, discussing what she and her mother were planning to do after the session and assuring her that the missed activities would be carried over to the next session. However, when the time came for the session to end, Amal was extremely upset, cried and repeatedly insisted for all the activities to be completed. The therapist calmly explained to Amal that unfortunately the session had to end, which led to a further discussion that schedules were useful to help plan activities or one's day. However, things happen unexpectedly, which means we cannot adhere to schedules rigidly. The therapist linked this to the ability to have flexible thinking patterns to help us remain regulated, or return to a state of feeling regulated or "just right". When the same happened a few sessions later, Amal was still upset but her reaction was less explosive, and she adapted more quickly to the change. Her mother also started working with her at home to develop daily schedules but took care to discuss with her what she could do, and how she could adapt when things did not go to plan.

When the therapist started exploring unhelpful thought patterns with Amal, it became apparent that these, perhaps more than her sensory processing differences, were contributing to her frequent emotional outbursts. As with the sensory-based concepts, Amal quickly understood the types of thought patterns that could influence her regulation states. However, Amal had significant difficulty personalising concepts and would frequently have emotional outbursts followed by crawling into her mother's lap and crying. The therapist kept her approach to Amal neutral during these times, and calmly described the behaviours she was seeing in relation to the concepts being taught. For example, when exploring different types of problem scenarios (some general and some specific to Amal that had been provided by her parents), Amal had difficulty accepting some problems that she viewed as hard or complex were actually "easy". On further probing, it became clear she thought that problems being classified as easy meant they were unimportant and had to be ignored, but she later understood this was not the case and that understanding the type of problem she was facing could help her solve the problem herself or "call in" the help of an adult such as her mother or teacher. Also, during a discussion on the possible motives of a classmate who often pulled her hair and called her names, Amal was adamant that the classmate was just "nasty". She did not want to accept another possible reason for her classmate's behaviour, such as that the classmate wanted to get her attention (although inappropriately) to play with her. Amal argued there was no way the therapist could know this, but the therapist gave the counter argument that in the same way there was no way Amal could know the girl was just trying to be nasty.

Amal still had some way to go to develop more helpful thought patterns to help with her ability to self-regulate, but her mother reported that her emotional outbursts were significantly reduced and they felt therapy provided her with better tools to help herself. Her parents reported the therapy she received was, "One of the most helpful things we have done to help Amal".

CASE STUDY 4: LLOYD

Background

Lloyd was a ten-year-old boy who loved science and any toys and games that had a building and construction element and which required problem solving. He was empathetic towards others and animals and had a strong sense of right and wrong. However, he often became overly anxious when he perceived things were "not right", and his parents reported he had significant difficulty coping when situations were not as he wanted them to be. He also struggled to accept anyone else's point regarding situations, as well as to accept constructive criticism. This often led to Lloyd having "emotional outbursts" and being verbally and/or physically aggressive towards others, and he often got into altercations with his peers. Following episodes of emotional outbursts, Lloyd would feel very upset and promised "not to do it again", although he did not have the skill set to change his behaviour accordingly. Furthermore, Lloyd's parents reported that he struggled coping with change, that he was impulsive with difficulties to concentrate, and that he had low self-confidence.

Before seeing an occupational therapist, Lloyd had been assessed by an educational psychologist as well as a consultant child and adolescent psychiatrist and clinical psychologist who together confirmed he had extremely high intelligence, attention deficit hyperactivity disorder or ADHD (for which he was taking medication during school time) and severe emotional regulation difficulties affecting his relationship with his peers. Lloyd also had a condition or malformation where brain tissue extends into the spinal canal. Effects vary from person to person with Lloyd experiencing shaky hands since he was young, resulting in his handwriting appearing messy. In an effort to better control his pen and subsequently produce neater handwriting, Lloyd would exert added pressure on the pen which caused him to experience pain in his writing hand after only short periods of writing.

Lloyd was one of a twin with his sibling having special needs since birth. This required frequent hospital and medical appointments, which Lloyd had to attend with his sibling and mother when he was younger, due to his father working abroad for extended periods of time. The educational psychologist had suggested that these unavoidable early family stressors had an impact on Lloyd's emotional development.

When Lloyd started with occupational therapy, he was attending a small weekly social emotional group at school aimed at developing coping strategies and appropriate behaviour in a variety of social situations, but his parents did not feel he was making a significant improvement. Lloyd had check-in sessions with a dedicated teacher at school, and they often took the school's therapy dog for regular walks on the school grounds. Lloyd was also attending weekly sessions at a local equestrian centre that specialised in supporting children with a variety of needs, which he enjoyed a lot.

Lloyd's parents' main concern and goal for therapy was that they wanted him to develop better emotional self-regulation skills so he could deal more effectively with the negative aspects of his life. When speaking with Lloyd himself, he confirmed he wanted to deal with situations better, although he told his mother he was not sure working with the occupational therapist would help, as "many others have tried already".

Main occupational therapy assessment findings

The occupational therapy assessment consisted both of a formal assessment and a class observation. The assessment confirmed Lloyd had difficulties with fine motor skills, which were thought to be partially related to his shaky hands. This was noticeable in the legibility of his handwriting and in his difficulty in writing for sustained periods without experiencing pain. This was reflected in his below average score for handwriting speed when tested using the DASH[3].

Lloyd had sensory processing differences and unhelpful thought patterns which contributed to some of his negative behaviours and emotional outbursts. Lloyd was sensitive to noise, which impacted on his ability to concentrate. Even when taking his ADHD medication, his ability to focus reduced significantly when working in noisy environments as opposed to quiet environments. He had reduced registration of visual stimuli, which meant he sometimes missed written instructions or struggled to find objects that were right in front of him. Lloyd needed to touch objects and people more than others, which caused his peers to be annoyed with him. However, he was sensitive to food textures and was described as a "picky eater", and he also had a reduced appetite because of his ADHD medication. Lloyd needed to move and fidget noticeably more than others, which is typical for a person with ADHD. Although he had responded well to medication, the occupational therapist could not rule out sensory processing differences as a contributory factor to his increased need for movement.

Lloyd displayed many of the characteristics common to children with high learning potential, most noticeably compassion for others, concerns with justice and fairness and emotional sensitivity. However, combined with inflexible thinking patterns, it was hard for him to understand other people's motives or accept their point of view, which in turn affected his self-esteem and contributed to his emotional outbursts.

When Lloyd was focussed, he seemed to easily understand and cope with academic work, but he often complained of feeling bored in class. The occupational therapist therefore agreed with the advice of the consultant child and adolescent psychiatrist and clinical psychologist that some of his fidgety behaviours were linked to intellectual boredom, and that his educators needed to consider continually giving him a higher level of challenge in academic work in order for him to remain engaged and motivated. Lloyd's school SENDCo also reported that he did much better in some teachers' classes than others, which the SENDCo attributed to the teaching style of the educators. Lloyd thrived more with teachers who were understanding, nurturing and able to "ignore" minor negative behaviour in class, but who were also able to give him clear structure and expectations of tasks he needed to complete.

The occupational therapist was of the opinion that there were multiple factors contributing to Lloyd's difficulties as described above, but also that he was gravely misunderstood by some of his educators and peers. Therefore, although Lloyd needed to develop appropriate emotional self-regulation skills, the therapist was of the opinion that his educators would also benefit from increased understanding of his complex profile and needs.

Stop! Consider and write down how you would approach working with Lloyd, keeping the 10 Golden Nuggets and 4 Essential Components in mind.

Therapy provision and outcome

Following the assessment, the therapist encouraged Lloyd's parents to meet with his school SENDCo and form teacher, in order to discuss the results and recommendations of the assessment. Among other things, the school needed to consider allowing Lloyd extra time when writing exams and supporting him to learn how to touch-type, in order to eventually be able to use a laptop for most of his writing tasks in school. Also, the therapist suggested more collaborative working between his teachers to better understand the approaches he responded to best.

Due to Lloyd's difficulties with focus and concentration, the occupational therapist suggested individual therapy sessions of 45 minutes each. However, as Lloyd was not sure whether therapy would help, the therapist agreed with him that they would do an initial three sessions, and thereafter he could decide whether he wanted to continue with therapy.

During the first three therapy sessions, Lloyd caught onto concepts very quickly and he reported that he enjoyed them and would like to continue with therapy. However, in a session not long after, Lloyd seemed oppositional and disengaged and would not respond to his mother's requests to focus during the session. It was confirmed that he had taken his ADHD medication and, according to his mother, he would normally be able to focus in these circumstances. Lloyd's mother became increasingly upset, and it led to a disagreement between them, which his mother explained happened often. The occupational therapist calmly explained to Lloyd what she perceived to be his mother's feelings in response to his observed behaviour, which his mother confirmed. The therapist also gave possible reasons for Lloyd's behaviour, these being that perhaps he was genuinely distracted, tired and/or that he did not really want to have therapy. Lloyd stated he was just tired, that he felt he benefited from therapy and that he had had no idea his behaviour had that effect on his mother.

The above led to a helpful discussion on how our behaviours, while with no ill-intent, can contribute to others misunderstanding and responding negatively to us. The therapist encouraged Lloyd and his mother to have more open communication between them, where they shared their feelings and thoughts when they had disagreements. While this did not address the wider issue of peer relationships, the therapist viewed it as a starting point for this. Also, the therapist had a separate discussion with Lloyd during which he stated he did not want to upset his mother during sessions, so the therapist suggested his mother not attend future sessions and only read the session summaries, to which he agreed. Lloyd's participation in sessions improved after this.

Even though Lloyd caught onto concepts quickly in therapy, he struggled to complete the occupational therapy homework between sessions. This was because of the family's full schedule and the pressures on his mother to manage the schedules of both Lloyd and his sibling, who attended a different school and continued to have hospital and therapy appointments. However, Lloyd agreed to read through the session summaries the therapist sent to his parents after sessions.

During the session in which the therapist discussed the auditory system, Lloyd reported he became extremely anxious when he heard buzzing insects. Lloyd described how he would cover his ears and run away, sometimes being teased by his peers about it. The school Lloyd attended was in a rural area with a lot of plants, trees and insect life, so this happened regularly. Lloyd told the therapist he was increasingly worried he was developing a phobia, but the therapist was able to explain to him it was his brain's natural response to sounds from the environment and he was more sensitive to noise than his peers. The therapist and Lloyd then brainstormed both thinking and sensory strategies to address this. Lloyd was able to change his perception about why he reacted the way he did, and instead of saying to himself, "I am developing a phobia", he replaced it with, "This is normal for me, but I can control my response". He also chose to do some quick proprioceptive-based activities or "calming exercises" when he heard buzzing insects, instead of acting on the urge to run away. Soon after, Lloyd's mother reported they had had an incident in the car where an insect was trapped. Instead of Lloyd reacting frantically, he stayed calm and did his exercises until the insect was out of the car.

When addressing unhelpful thought patterns, Lloyd found it easy to write down what his "cloudy voice" was saying to him in situations, but he found it exceptionally hard to activate the cloudy voice's opposite "sunny voice" for the same situations. The therapist took care to encourage Lloyd to identify his cloudy voice in challenging situations and activate the sunny voice. Lloyd started improving in this area, although the therapist anticipated it would be an ongoing process.

During the time Lloyd was receiving occupational therapy, he decided with his parents that he needed a more structured schooling environment, and he was successful in his application to a military boarding school in England. Towards the end of therapy, the therapist arranged a meeting with Lloyd's parents during which they discussed how his parents could support him in his new school, such as meeting with the school SENDCo beforehand to discuss his needs, both in terms of his high learning potential and also his ADHD and sensory processing differences. The therapist also talked about the "big change" with Lloyd, and they brainstormed some coping strategies he could use to help him. The therapist offered to write a home program for him, but he had already started to work through a book called *Thriving With ADHD Workbook For Kids: 60 Fun Activities to Help Children Self-Regulate, Focus and Succeed* by Kelli Miller. The therapist and Lloyd discussed some of the book's content, and he was able to draw comparisons with the concepts they had encountered in therapy. So, they agreed he would complete the workbook instead.

At the end of therapy, Lloyd's parents reported they were fully satisfied with the process and its results. They stated,

> From the beginning of therapy, we have been able to talk with Lloyd about what might work best for him (and us), and the sense of participation (from the therapist) was a tremendous help in understanding how we might help Lloyd. He appeared to pick up on the ethos of the sessions and, at least, in the immediate time after each session he was clearly more able to apply control when feeling anxious/angry/frustrated.

A year after therapy ended, Lloyd's parents got in touch with the therapist to report on his progress. They stated he had settled well into his new school, and they felt he benefited from the routine and organised structure it provided, receiving almost no negative feedback regarding his behaviour. Lloyd was also doing well academically, being first in his class for French and geography, and with his extra curricular activities such as preparing for his first public concert playing an instrument. Overall, Lloyd's parents reported he was doing much better with managing his emotions since receiving occupational therapy; although he still struggled in this area particularly when he was at home where family life was often unpredictable. However, they mentioned they often had to remind themselves he was still young and he had come far in a short space of time.

CASE STUDY 5: IMOGEN

Background

Imogen was a thirteen-year-old girl (Year 9 in England and Wales) with confirmed high learning potential. Her parents described her as very academic, a good communicator, especially at debating, curious about the world and creative. She enjoyed reading historical fiction books and watching historical documentaries, writing plays, baking and making things, and attended regular ice skating lessons. However, she had severe anxieties about attending school, was constantly "on edge" and unable to relax, and experienced intense frustration and anger about the world. She was also very disorganised and struggled with some everyday motor skills tasks, such as eating awkwardly with cutlery and frequently bumping into others and objects. Imogen had low self-esteem and was very critical of herself and sometimes others, showing strong perfectionistic traits. She felt she was very different to and mentally more mature than her peers. Although she had a few friends, on the whole she struggled to form friendships as she was of the opinion that others did not want to be friends with her, and she responded very strongly when teased by them.

At the time Imogen's parents requested occupational therapy, she was also awaiting an assessment by a psychologist from the Children and Adolescent Mental Health Services (CAMHS) for anxiety and obsessive compulsive behaviours. Imogen's parents thought she could benefit from occupational therapy to help her relax, calm down and feel happier in general.

Main occupational therapy assessment findings

Imogen was keen to get help for her difficulties, but was unsure about occupational therapy as she had never heard about it before. The therapist offered to first meet with her and her mother to have an informal discussion about how occupational therapy could help, which she was happy to do. After this initial meeting, Imogen felt she wanted to engage with occupational therapy. During the full assessment, she put maximum effort into all the tasks and activities presented, and during a free-writing task, she wrote an exceptional piece on the evolution of fashion during the Victorian era.

The occupational therapy assessment highlighted that Imogen had sensory processing differences and possibly an inherent motor coordination difficulty. She had already taught herself some adequate strategies for new and unfamiliar motor tasks, such as analysing the tasks and "talking herself through" them. With regards to her sensory profile, Imogen was particularly sensitive to and got distracted by noisy environments. She became very anxious when standing close to others, but also needed to touch textures and surfaces more than others and was constantly fiddling with her hands or chewing on pens to the point of breaking them. Imogen needed to move much more than her peers, and had difficulties judging the correct force when doing tasks and when mobilising, describing herself as "heavy footed".

Imogen had some unhelpful thought patterns that were contributing to her anxiety levels, the most notable being that she continually placed extreme pressure on herself to score top marks in all of her tests as she felt that anything less would result in her not being able to study a course at university some day. When she did not achieve top marks, Imogen felt disappointed and scolded herself, further impacting on her low self-esteem.

Stop! Consider and write down how you would approach working with Imogen, keeping the 10 Golden Nuggets and 4 Essential Components in mind.

Therapy provision and outcome

Following the occupational therapy assessment, the therapist had a meeting with Imogen and her mother, during which they discussed the assessment results at length. Imogen asked many questions about her assessed motor and sensory needs and the root causes for these and expressed her relief upon learning there were reasons for some of her difficulties. The therapist asked Imogen what she wanted to work on, and she responded that she still felt exploring how to deal with her sensory and thought environments were the most important to her at that time. The therapist explained the overall progression of therapy and that she was anticipating some sessions would be harder for Imogen than others. However, the therapist assured Imogen that she was in control of her therapy progression, and that she could ask for a break in therapy, or for therapy to stop at any point if she wanted to.

There was a delay of a few weeks before Imogen started occupational therapy, as her mental health deteriorated and her anxieties around attending school spiked. She was getting to school later each day, began refusing to do any type of writing and her behaviour at home became labile. At this time, she started seeing a psychologist from CAMHS who diagnosed her with obsessive compulsive disorder and who recommended she consider taking medication and receiving cognitive behavioural therapy. Imogen and her mother discussed the possibility of occupational therapy alongside the psychologist's input and asked whether the psychologist had any concerns about both therapies happening simultaneously, but the psychologist welcomed it and so did the occupational therapist. Imogen was also taken under the care of a psychiatrist to prescribe and manage her medication.

Imogen attended five double occupational therapy sessions, each of one-and-a-half hours, alongside her sessions with the psychologist. Her mother was present for all sessions. During this time, her anxieties and obsessive compulsive thought patterns and behaviours intensified, and she started hitting her head randomly throughout the day to get rid of the fearful thoughts that she was losing her intellectual abilities. Together with her parents and school, it was decided she would not attend school so she could focus on her mental health. She also declined from meeting with her friends or going ice skating.

Imogen looked forward to occupational therapy sessions but refused to write at all. The therapist adapted sessions and homework so that Imogen could "direct" her or her mother who scribed for her. Imogen benefitted from discussing the concepts she was learning in therapy at length and also reported on the management strategies she was learning about in her psychology sessions, which she also did in her psychology sessions with regards to her occupational therapy strategies. Imogen was able to draw comparisons on how the therapies complemented each other and which strategies she could use in various situations; this was enhanced by Imogen gaining further insight into her feelings and behaviours by keeping a diary for a couple of days.

When discussing different types of self-talk, Imogen initially argued that a person's negative and positive self-talk or "voices" could not be separated and had the same purpose of propelling one to perfection, such as needing to get top marks in tests. The therapist calmly challenged this thought pattern and, by giving practical examples of the different effects of negative and positive self-talk on a person's self-esteem and motivation to participate in activities, Imogen conceded they were different and she saw the value of developing her positive self-talk more. She also enjoyed creating different objects with play dough as a means to understand she needed to develop her flexible thinking alongside her positive self-talk. She agreed that a trusted adult who understood these concepts, such as her mother, could point out negative self-talk and inflexible thought patterns as and when they appeared to occur, and that they could work together to "activate the opposites".

Imogen started attending some of her ice skating lessons again, and towards the end of therapy, she went to an indoor trampoline park, and she also attempted to write a few words. Her mother reported that she asked to go back to school soon after, and her school was very supportive in implementing a phased return to school. She managed to attend school for an increasing number of hours each day for a period of two weeks, but all schools then closed across England due to the Covid 19 national lockdowns.

The family stayed in touch with the therapist, and a few months later her mother reported the lockdowns had benefited Imogen, stating she had, worked hard for the whole of lockdown, completing lots of school assignments.

She also spent time doing things that hadn't been possible for a while - gardening, painting, baking bread and cake, sewing, learning how to use the washing machine. She also decided to enter an historical fiction writing competition. She wrote 18,000 words, which was so exciting after she had been unable to write. She is now more open minded about how the future might unfold. She has also been doing some exercise and movement each day. She is very determined to make a good start to Year 10, so fingers crossed.

CASE STUDY 6: THEO

Background

Theo was a six-year-old boy with suspected high learning potential. He was a happy boy and had an extensive vocabulary considering his age. Theo had a wide range of interests, loved learning how to read and was very imaginative; he relished making up stories as he played. He had two brothers, one seven years old and the other three years old, and his mother was a teacher by background who home educated the children. They also attended various other educational groups during the week, such as forest school where Theo loved collecting bugs.

Theo had sensory processing differences, and the occupational therapist had worked with him two years prior, helping his parents understand his needs and learning about activities to help him regulate, which were effective at the time. However, as Theo grew and his personality and imaginational overexcitabilities developed, he was reluctant to engage in sensory-based activities merely on his parents' suggestion.

Theo's parents reported he was particularly sensitive to noise, such as his younger brother crying, and he had a definite need to touch others and objects more than others his age. Theo was generally very active, but not always productive or regulated, which not only affected his learning and development, but also his relationships with his brothers and peers. For example, he loved doing mental maths, playing word games, playing strategic as well as chance-based board games, completing workbooks or doing crafts at the table for hours. These all whilst standing and moving around, which was not considered to be a problem. Theo also had a wobble cushion for his seat at the dinner table, but he preferred to stand or walk around during meal times. However, he seemed to be increasingly in a state of "dysregulation" during which he climbed on people, especially his brothers, pushed his feet into people or pulled on their arms, which upset them. He would do so without understanding that his behaviour was considered inappropriate. Theo would roll on the floor, push his head into the sofa, bounce on furniture, throw objects around and get upset over tiny things, resulting in him screaming and hitting others. This caused his parents to have to separate him from his brothers for safety reasons, which he also found very upsetting. Theo's parents

184 *Case Studies*

described his episodes of dysregulation as him being "over excited", during which he would also not respond to them and avoid all eye contact.

Theo seemed to be calmer when outdoors, but his behaviour when going on outings was unpredictable, with the family often having to return early from educational trips such as visiting museums. However, they had found there was a better chance of success if Theo could learn at his own pace through self-directed exploration of museums or similar educational venues and engage in hands-on or play-based activities as opposed to "listening" to others' teaching.

Theo's parents wanted him to engage in further occupational therapy, in order for him to gain an understanding of his own regulation states and needs and how to meet these himself, due to not responding to others' input.

Main occupational therapy assessment findings

The occupational therapy assessment confirmed Theo's sensory processing differences, and that his motor skills were average for his age group. Theo also scored particularly highly in visual perceptual and visual motor integrative abilities. During the assessment the therapist had to repeat instructions several times as Theo seemed to process auditory information slower than expected and also struggled to keep more than one instruction in his head at a time. This affected his ability to organise himself significantly. Furthermore, Theo's speech production was slow and not always clear, and he would often repeat the first word of a sentence until he could "find" the rest of the words to describe something, which he then did in detail.

Stop! Consider and write down how you would approach working with Theo, keeping the 10 Golden Nuggets and 4 Essential Components in mind.

Therapy provision and outcome

Occupational therapy sessions aimed at helping Theo develop increased self awareness and management strategies to help his difficulties with self-regulation were suggested. The therapist also recommended that Theo's parents consider an assessment by a speech and language therapist to determine whether his speech and language development, in particular his speech/sound production, was as expected, and to provide input as appropriate. In addition, the therapist suggested that an assessment by a child psychiatrist/psychologist/paediatrician would be appropriate in order to confirm or rule out an attention disorder and to provide advice as appropriate.

Theo attended five double therapy sessions, with his mother present during all sessions. Sessions were as practical and "hands on" as possible, and the therapist presented activities at Theo's pace, repeating sentences as necessary to accommodate for his observed slow auditory processing. However, Theo caught onto all the concepts being taught very quickly and could explore the ones that interested him most in more depth. He particularly enjoyed exploring developing a language to describe his different states of regulation. As his parents often referred to his state of dysregulation as him being "over excited", some further discussion was needed around the difference between being excited but still able to "do what you have to do" and being excited but unable "do what you have to do". For example, Theo realised it was positive for him to become very excited during forest school when he found bugs and yet still be able to learn more about them (regulated state), but it was negative when he became very excited to the point where it felt like he wanted to pull on his brothers' arms and climb all over them, which resulted in them being upset and fighting with him (dysregulated state). He understood that during such times he needed to consider strategies to help feel calmer, become more regulated and avoid negative behaviour and upset. The occupational therapist made a point of frequently also describing her own feelings, whether in response to a sensory need or thought pattern, e.g. "I feel a little tired today so did a few bounces on the mini trampoline before you came to help me feel more awake and ready for our session", or, "the noise from that lawn mower outside is bothering my ears and makes me feel agitated, so I may need to ask for some 'time out' to do a few deep breathing exercises when I feel the noise starting to make me angry".

Theo benefitted from keeping a diary with his mother of the activities he did over a period of three non-consecutive days. When discussing this with the therapist, he could recognise the pattern for activities where he felt regulated, and the ones where he did not. This motivated him to regularly draw up with his mother a simple schedule of the activities planned for the next day, and helped him realise when he could engage in the sensory activities he was learning about to help him feel more alert or calm, depending on the demands of the activities.

As it was not clear why Theo sometimes became very upset about minor things, the therapist also explored various thinking patterns with him. He enjoyed learning about flexible and inflexible thinking patterns, as well as positive and negative self-talk, but it became apparent he did not struggle significantly in these areas, so the therapist did not spend much time exploring these concepts in detail with him. However, Theo benefitted from discovering how the classification of problems could assist with the speed of solving them, particularly in relation to his siblings. For example, Theo gained insight into the fact that the discomfort he felt when his younger brother cried was in fact an easy problem to resolve as it was "simple, well understood, required little thought and could be solved easily and/or quickly" (see Chapter 7, Table 7.5. Thought Environment: Common Types of Thought Patterns and Suggested Exploration Activities, Concern with Justice and Fairness, Preoccupation with Problems Often Affecting Activity Participation, but with Associated Drive to Solve Problems).

In other words, the crying was a noise that hurt his ears and made him feel "over excited" (simple/well understood/required little thought once identified), and he could deal with this by covering his ears and/or putting on ear defenders and/or going into another room with a safe sensory space to help him feel calmer (could be solved easily and/or quickly). Theo and his mother agreed to construct a themed sensory den in one of their rooms with some sensory-based activities and equipment to help him feel calmer, such as ear defenders, therapy putty and dragon colouring sheets, already set up. The theme would be on one of the many stories Theo made up. At one point during the discussion on types of problems, Theo had an "aha moment" and said, "Now, that is very helpful!"

At the end of therapy, Theo's mother reported,

> Theo enjoyed all his therapy sessions. The therapist took things at his pace, responding to his needs as she saw them arise and always looked for the reason behind his behaviours rather than hurrying him through activities or telling him to stop. The therapist helped me really understand his sensory needs and the many strategies I can use to support him. The sessions have helped me have realistic expectations of him and enable him to achieve these. The therapist has also helped Theo begin to understand his own needs, and this is very helpful as we can now talk to him about his states of regulation, and also if and how he needs to change them. We are so thankful for this input!

CASE STUDY 7: LUCAS

Background

Lucas was a seven-year-old boy (Year 2 in England and Wales) with confirmed high learning potential, which was evident from the moment anyone met him. He had a highly developed vocabulary, a keen sense of humour and enjoyed wordplay, loved reading books beyond his expected age level and read for hours on end. Lucas had a particular talent for maths, and when tested had scored at the level of Year 6 (ten to 11 years old) in this area. He was also becoming interested in chess and was focussed on developing his skills in this area. Lucas was very curious about the world and regularly invented elaborate but well-defined schemes and plans, such as for high-tech hide outs for him and his friends. He was comfortable in his own company and preferred having a small group of friends. He also enjoyed being active outdoors.

Lucas's parents requested occupational therapy on the advice of an educational psychologist as they wanted to know how to further support him. Their main concerns were that he sometimes struggled with his emotions, which resulted in distress and emotional outbursts about small issues. They also felt he lacked some self-confidence and seemed insecure despite being proud of his abilities, and that his social skills were variable and not in line with his developed cognitive abilities. They hoped occupational therapy would help them gain a better understanding of Lucas's strengths and weaknesses and provide him with the strategies to cope when he found things difficult.

Main occupational therapy assessment findings

The occupational therapist carried out a full assessment with Lucas, during which he seemed very interested in each new activity and was keen to do them to the best of his ability. Lucas discussed his advanced abilities in maths, and therefore asked for his motor skills to be assessed at the higher age band too but agreed to be tested at his age level. When the therapist analysed all the information from the assessment, his motor skills were found to be below average for his age and in line with the features of developmental coordination disorder. This was supported by his reported and observed difficulties with other motor-based tasks, such as writing legibly, catching a ball and riding a bicycle without stabilisers.

Lucas often stated he found school very boring, but his parents found this confusing as he would often ask for maths work to be presented at an advanced level, but for other work to be at reception level (age four equivalent). He also sometimes stated that in class he struggled with maths, but on further discussion it became clear he was referring to the cutting and sticking of shapes rather than the subject itself. It also transpired his teacher would keep children who did not finish these tasks in class during break time to finish them, so Lucas developed the habit of rushing said tasks, which reduced the quality of his work.

Furthermore, Lucas had some sensory processing differences, with a mixed sensory profile. He was highly sensitive to unexpected noise, which was indicative of a retained Moro reflex. He also had other retained reflexes which impacted his seated posture. He needed to move much more than his peers, which presented as frequently approaching his teacher and often fiddling with objects to the annoyance of others. Lucas was sensitive to having messy hands and would avoid activities that required his hands getting dirty.

Personality-wise, Lucas was very motivated to succeed at whatever tasks he engaged with, he had high expectations of himself with strong perfectionistic traits, was competitive and had wonderful ideas of how to adapt games with his peers to make them more interesting. However, he did not understand why his friends did not want to follow his suggestions and struggled to accept games played on their terms.

The therapist concluded that Lucas displayed the profile of DME/2e. He had asynchronous development borne out of his advanced abilities in maths and reading and delayed motor skills, which sometimes impacted on what he was able to "produce" in subjects. Also, he had advanced cognitive abilities and imaginational overexcitabilities, but his emotional development was not advanced to the same degree, although not necessarily lagging behind his peers. Lucas expected all of his abilities to be at the same level as his cognitive abilities, but he also had some awareness that he was struggling in some areas, though he could not determine the reasons for this. The therapist hypothesised that all the factors mentioned above contributed to Lucas's emotional outbursts, lack of self-confidence and feelings of insecurity and variable social skills.

Stop! Consider and write down how you would approach working with Lucas, keeping the 10 Golden Nuggets and 4 Essential Components in mind.

Therapy provision and outcome

The therapist discussed the results of the assessment thoroughly with Lucas's parents to help them gain a better understanding of his assessed needs. The therapist also recommended they schedule a meeting with the school SENDCo and Lucas's class teacher to discuss the report and help the school team to gain a better understanding of his strengths and challenges. To support this, the therapist also made some recommendations that could be implemented immediately in school, such as reviewing his table and chair set-up in class to ensure it promoted a good seated position, for Lucas to be allowed short but purposeful sensory breaks in the classroom, to be given hand gloves for activities that required his hands to get messy or for him to be allowed to participate in an alternative way and for teachers to ensure he heard and understood instructions when given in a noisy environment.

The therapist suggested occupational therapy to initially focus on helping Lucas with his motor skills, specifically to do reflex integration exercises at home, and to develop adequate scissor cutting skills in therapy to support his maths lessons and to then move on to helping him develop increased self-awareness in his sensory and thought environments, which he seemed very excited about. Lucas responded very well to the first three single sessions aimed at improving his scissor cutting skills. The therapist chose activities in which he was required to cut out templates of 3D shapes, and then stick them together, using principles from the Cognitive Orientation to Daily Occupational Performance (CO-OP/CO-OP Approach)™ to help him analyse and adjust his performance. Lucas practised hard between sessions and was happy with his improvement.

Therapy then shifted to addressing Lucas's sensory and thought environments using the DME-C approach. Lucas started with two double sessions aimed at developing a language to describe feelings, and that introduced the different types of sensory stimuli and thought patterns that could help him feel more regulated. Lucas enjoyed the novelty of the activities but did not do the related therapy homework between the first and second double sessions, stating he did not see the point when asked. He also seemed noticeably disengaged in the second double session and said it was because he was tired. The therapist agreed with Lucas and his mother that the next session would be a single session, but during this session Lucas was even more disengaged. This led to the therapist having an open discussion with Lucas about how he really felt about therapy, assuring him that he would not get in trouble if he shared his real thoughts, but that it was important to know as he was an equal partner in the therapy process. Lucas admitted he felt he benefited from therapy, but only because it meant he missed "boring school". The therapist objectively analysed the situation and gave Lucas the option to stop therapy altogether, coming back if and when he felt he needed it, to which he agreed.

Lucas's parents were disappointed that he did not want to continue with therapy, but understood he had to be internally motivated to work on his sensory and thought environments for therapy to be successful. During a debriefing session, Lucas's parents agreed they felt the occupational therapy already provided had helped them gain better insight into his needs, how to support him and how to advocate for him.

Note from authors: We have included this case study in the book to show therapists that, despite having a "child with a clear DME/2e profile", it is important to regularly analyse the effectiveness of input being provided. Therapists should be prepared to make adaptations to therapy as needed to best help the child, even if it means stopping therapy for a period of time or altogether.

CASE STUDY 8: ANDY

Background

Andy was a thirteen-year-old boy with confirmed high learning potential and lived with his parents and younger sibling. His parents described him as buzzing with mental energy, being very enthusiastic and interested in a range of topics such as science, politics, current affairs, religion and philosophy. Andy liked sci-fi books and films and played lots of computer games requiring creativity in various ways. He also enjoyed being active but preferred participating in parkour* due to its freestyle nature, instead of traditional sports that were rules-based and/or competitive. Andy was a very engaging person and his parents enjoyed talking and going places with him.

Prior to working with the occupational therapist, Andy had already been identified as having behavioural, emotional and social development difficulties. He had a history of struggling to cope in school environments and had been excluded from two schools, one which specialised in helping children with said difficulties. Andy had an Educational and Health Care Plan (EHCP)† in place, and when the occupational therapist met him, he was doing an online home education program as part of an agreement with his local educational authority to meet his learning needs, which his parents reported suited him well. He also received dramatherapy and responded positively according to his parents.

Andy's parents' ongoing concerns were that he had significant emotional reactions to failure or when feeling frustrated, that he struggled to meet social norms, and that he had sensory processing differences and motor skills difficulties that affected his everyday life. For example, he felt very different from his peers and struggled to interact with them, which was exacerbated by the fact that he had been bullied and teased. Andy struggled to settle at night and go to sleep, became easily overwhelmed in noisy environments or during long car journeys, struggled to eat with cutlery and was very disorganised apart from when he engaged in academic work, which he seemed to approach in systematic ways. Andy had struggled with his mental health in the past, and was known to his local Children and Adolescent Mental Health Services (CAMHS). He had also previously received occupational therapy to address his sensory needs.

Andy and his parents' main goal for therapy was for him to better understand the interaction between his emotional, sensory and social needs and to develop appropriate coping strategies and social skills.

Main occupational therapy assessment findings

Andy's occupational therapy assessment confirmed that he had sensory processing differences, with an overall profile of being sensitive to and avoidant of noise, bright lights and certain food textures. Andy also displayed proprioceptive seeking behaviour more than his peers, such as frequently needing to stretch his legs or "squeeze" his muscles, which was noticeable during car journeys. Andy's motor skills and general disorganised state were in line with the features of developmental coordination disorder. Furthermore, he had strong perfectionist traits, was very afraid of making mistakes and had inflexible thinking patterns with regards to the motives of others in social situations. All of these challenges combined to negatively impact Andy's self-esteem, social emotional responses and activity participation.

Stop! Consider and write down how you would approach working with Andy, keeping the 10 Golden Nuggets and 4 Essential Components in mind.

Therapy provision and outcome

Andy had a range of identified occupational therapy needs, but when his parents discussed the assessment results with him, he confirmed that he was most motivated to work on managing the interactions between his sensory, emotional and social needs. Andy attended five double therapy sessions, each of one-and-a-half hours and with one of his parents present. His father benefited greatly from attending sessions and became very excited at learning about the concepts and how to help Andy, but also plainly stated that for the first time in his own life he understood himself better, as he and Andy shared many of the same traits.

Andy understood concepts with regards to both his sensory and thought environments exceptionally quickly and almost always adapted them to make them more relevant to him. For example, when discussing the use of colours as a way to describe his feelings, he chose the colours purple to represent the overall feelings of being sad or stressed, green with the overall feelings of calm, happy and focussed, red with the feeling of losing control, and black with the overall feelings of angry, annoyed and excited. Also, when given the options of how he would like to keep a diary of the main activities he was engaged in over a few days and how they made him feel, Andy said he would, "take it away and think about it". Andy came back to the following session, having written down his activities in paragraph style, numbering each main activity and how it made him feel. For example,

> Thursday. Number one, I woke up and felt pretty tired since I read quite late into the night. Number two, Ate breakfast and played with therapy putty, which woke me up. Number three, Did maths and played with the therapy putty again, which made me happier and raised my energy level. Number four, Did English, which was boring, so I felt slower. Number five, Did science then ate lunch which cheered me up a little. Number six, Did history, but before this I felt a little bored so it kind of carried over. Number seven, Did parkour which was quite exciting and made me feel very tired afterwards. Number eight, Had supper, Indian, which cheered me up. Number nine, Went to bed, but felt way too hot, so I got upset and angry. Took a shower, then went back to bed again.

As Andy and his father learnt about the principles of managing his sensory needs, they had lots of lively discussions and "aha" moments. As a result, Andy was curious to know about as many sensory-based activities as he could to help him regulate better. Therefore, instead of asking him to discover specific activities on his own between sessions, the therapist decided to give Andy a list of everyday sensory activities, which he agreed to try at home under the supervision of his parents in order to decide if he wanted to use them. Andy ended up with quite an extensive list, but needed reminding to purposefully choose only a few to use in specific situations and/or those he anticipated to be stressful.

Andy advised the therapist that although he struggled with repetitive background noise such as the ticking of a wall clock, he preferred and was focussed when doing homework with music that was loud and had a strong beat. Andy was surprised to realise he became distressed when looking at bright lights and could think of ways to address this. He already knew he had a strong aversion to certain food textures, but was happy to explore whether there were healthy food and drink options he could use to help him regulate better. Andy particularly enjoyed learning about activities he could use during car journeys, such as placing a theraband[‡] under his feet and pulling up on the sides with his hands, sitting on his hands, doing deep breathing and playing with resistive toys such as a football fidget cube.

During the sessions in which the therapist discussed the types of thought patterns that seemed to influence him negatively, Andy was remarkably receptive to discussing these and "finding their opposites". Andy identified that he had recurrent negative self-talk whenever he wrote tests or sat in a car for long journeys along the lines of, "You are terrible, you are idiotic", and was able to activate the opposite positive self-talk such as, "You got this, you can do this". He also readily explored some of his inflexible thinking patterns with regards to his fear of making mistakes, as well as the motives of others when playing with him. Andy was able to analyse how inflexible thinking patterns may have contributed to some of his own frustrations and low self-esteem, as well as some of the disagreements he had in the past with his peers.

Towards the end of therapy, Andy and his parents informed the therapist they had found a visual brainstorming and mind mapping app which aims to help people connect their thoughts and clarify their ideas in a visual way. They were going to trial it as their next "project" to help Andy with his general disorganisation. When therapy ended, Andy and his parents told the therapist they felt sessions had really helped him and he had learnt a lot from the process. Andy did not request any follow up sessions, but his parents stayed in touch with the therapist, and three years later reported that,

> Andy really benefited from the occupational therapy support. He did some of his GCSEs[§] last year to not have too much pressure now, and is currently preparing to write the rest. He is also looking forward to a trip to Paris with a friend after he has completed his GCSEs, and is very excited about joining the sixth form in a local school in the new school year.

CASE STUDY 9: KELI

Background

Keli was an autistic eight-year-old boy (Year 4 in England and Wales), with high learning potential. He had an extensive general knowledge, read a wide variety of books and loved watching game shows on television. He also enjoyed participating in a variety of sports such as football (soccer), golf, tennis and basketball.

Keli's parents were concerned that he struggled to control his emotions and that he got angry very quickly. Keli had told his parents he wanted help to feel less worried and nervous about things all the time; and he also wanted to know how "he could be less fidgety" in school as he sometimes got into trouble in class. Keli's parents researched the possible help available and decided on occupational therapy. Both Keli and his parents were motivated for him to develop the skills and abilities to cope better with his emotions.

Main occupational therapy assessment findings

During the assessment, Keli told the occupational therapist he wanted to do things perfectly, and when he did not succeed in this he got angry, upset and felt like a failure. Keli's desire to carry out tasks perfectly was noticeable throughout the assessment and clearly affected his task participation. He approached all tasks with exceptional care and seemed to exert a high level of physical effort. At times Keli became visibly distressed when it appeared that he was not performing tasks "perfectly", and the therapist had to intervene and help him calm down.

With formal testing, Keli's motor skills fell within the normal range for his age. However, observations of the quality of his movements of everyday tasks by his parents and the occupational therapist, suggested he had a significant movement difficulty, specifically with regards to fine motor skills tasks such as eating with cutlery or tying his shoelaces. The assessment also confirmed that Keli had sensory processing differences, more specifically sensitivity to noise and an increased need for movement and heavy work. He often fiddled with objects and rocked on his chair in class to the point of falling off. The occupational therapist was of the opinion that Keli's difficulties with fine motor tasks and his sensory processing differences, combined with his desire for perfectionism, contributed to his intense feelings of frustration and anger when he did not perform tasks "perfectly", which in turn affected his ability to regulate his emotions appropriately.

Stop! Consider and write down how you would approach working with Keli, keeping the 10 Golden Nuggets and 4 Essential Components in mind.

Therapy provision and outcome

Directly following the occupational therapy assessment, the therapist spoke to Keli and asked him to remember the phrases "doing things perfectly" vs. "doing things with excellence" for when they started working together.

The therapist recommended that Keli's therapy firstly focussed on receiving help with regards to understanding and dealing with his sensory and thought environments following the principles of the DME-C approach; and thereafter on improving the motor skills tasks he was having difficulty with and wanted to work on, such as eating with cutlery and doing his shoe laces, by following principles of the Cognitive Orientation to Daily Occupational Performance (CO-OP/CO-OP Approach)™. Keli agreed to this course of action, and was very excited to work with the therapist. Keli attended five double therapy sessions of one-and-a-half hours each with his mother attending all sessions.

Keli easily understood the concepts with regards to his sensory environment, and his confidence seemed to grow with each session as he became more aware of his own sensory preferences as well as how he could use his senses to help him when he was struggling in noisy environments and with his general intense need for movement. Keli, his mother and the therapist had long discussions about the use of schedules, as this provided him with the necessary structure for when would be the most appropriate times to engage in his chosen sensory activities to help him feel more regulated. For example, Keli started understanding that doing movement and heavy work activities in the morning before school helped him to be less fidgety in class, specifically for morning lessons. His mother also stated that she was growing in her understanding of his specific needs and was proactive in meeting with Keli's school SENDCO after each therapy session to discuss the strategies he was learning and how it could be incorporated into his school day in an appropriate way.

When addressing the unhelpful thought patterns that were connected to Keli's anger and feelings of failure when he was unable to perform tasks perfectly, he benefited most from direct statements. For example, early on in the therapy program the therapist told Keli that it was okay not to be perfect. The therapist also told him that there was a difference between "doing things perfectly" and "doing things with excellence". Perfectionism was striving for the impossible, and it caused people to dwell on their mistakes which resulted in feelings of frustration and failure. In contrast, excellence was striving for the positive, and it caused people to learn from their mistakes, which resulted in feelings of fulfilment and success. The therapist also "dropped" these statements into various conversations throughout the course of therapy, such as during the "paper plate painting with salad spinner" activity where Keli tried very hard to produce the same painting as the therapist but did not succeed. Months after therapy had ended, Keli's mother got in touch with the therapist to report on a situation where Keli "failed". However, instead of getting angry, he told his mother, "Remember, it is okay not to be perfect!"

In addition to the above, Keli enjoyed learning about the different classification of problems and discussing possible solutions to a range of problems. This also helped him to identify when he could try and resolve it on his own and when he needed to call in the help of an adult such as his mother or sports coach.

When the first phase of therapy concluded, Keli and his parents stated they did not immediately want to continue with addressing his motor skills difficulties. Keli's parents reported that working with a professional who "got" their son's complex profile of high learning potential, autism and sensory needs was a relief. They felt that occupational therapy was "unique" and that the therapist "adapted to Keli's needs during every session, allowing him to be who he is". They stated that occupational therapy "supported him effectively", that he continued to use the sensory and thought based strategies he learnt during therapy, and that it had made a positive difference to his ability to manage his emotions more effectively.

CASE STUDY 10: MARCO

Background

Marco was a twelve-year-old boy in his first year of secondary school at an international bilingual school in England. He had high learning potential, an extensive vocabulary, enjoyed reading and participating in drama, and his favourite subject was history.

Marco's parents described that he was generally very boisterous, with a high need for movement, and emotionally intense. In primary school, Marco achieved top marks for most subjects without much effort, but he struggled more since starting secondary school, becoming very oppositional, mostly refusing to do homework and having regular emotional outbursts. Marco's parents reported he wanted to have lots of friends but he struggled with friendships. He did not get invited to many birthday parties, which they felt was because he came across as too bossy and he had a short temper. Marco therefore often "escaped" to his books during breaktime at school. However, he had attended a social skills development group when he started secondary school and since then had made some friends.

Marco's need for movement and fidgeting often got him into trouble at school as he was unable to "sit still" during lessons. He was also very intolerant to some smells and tastes and would seem highly irritated in food halls or similar environments. He also reacted aggressively when being touched by others.

Marco's parents requested occupational therapy, as they wanted to understand whether his behaviour was because of sensory processing differences and how they could support him. They also hoped therapy could help him develop appropriate management strategies for his difficulties.

Main occupational therapy assessment findings

Marco's overall behaviour during the assessment suggested he had many of the typical traits of children with high learning potential, but he had not yet been able to develop them to his advantage. Even though he had agreed to the assessment beforehand, he directly told the therapist upon arrival he did not want to be there. With encouragement, he agreed to participate and give maximum effort with the activities presented, but he labelled many of the activities as pointless or boring, generally rushing through them.

Although Marco approached most tasks with a seeming indifferent attitude, he appeared keen to do well in them. For example, when asked to write on a topic of his choice, which was history, he struggled to start as he said he wanted it to be very good on his first attempt. At other times, he refused to do the tasks altogether, stating that he could not do it and therefore was not even going to try. This demonstrated Marco's perfectionism and the high standards he set for himself, as well as his fear of failure.

Marco also displayed some inflexible thinking patterns during the assessment with regards to the motives of others, combined with immature emotional responses. For example, even though he knew how long the assessment was likely to take, he became very upset after the first hour when the therapist suggested they take a break and said that he felt tricked as he thought the assessment was over.

The assessment confirmed that Marco had sensory processing differences that were impacting on his activity participation and behaviour. Marco sought out movement and heavy work more than his peers, e.g. frequently not sitting still, finding endless reasons to approach the teacher and fiddling with objects or pushing his peers around the classroom. Marco displayed sensitivity towards strong smells such as coffee and tastes such as spicy food and tactile sensitivity such as being easily upset by minor injuries or reacting negatively when others touched him. However, he also displayed tactile sensory seeking behaviour such as touching people or objects to the point of annoyance. Marco also had reduced visual registration as he frequently needed help to find objects that were obvious to others and sometimes missed directions in class.

The occupational therapist was of the opinion that there were various factors contributing to Marco's difficulties as described above, and because these difficulties affected his behaviour over time, it led to him being generally misunderstood by others. In turn, this contributed to Marco having a highly developed sense of distrust when it came to authority figures. The therapist therefore felt that Marco's educators needed to also better understand his strengths, challenges and needs alongside any therapy he may receive.

Stop! Consider and write down how you would approach working with Marco, keeping the 10 Golden Nuggets and 4 Essential Components in mind.

Therapy provision and outcome

Directly following the occupational therapy assessment, the therapist spoke with Marco and his mother in a calm and non-judgmental way, stating that her initial thoughts were that, even though he was very bright, it did not appear his social and emotional skills had developed in line with his intellectual ability. The therapist explained to Marco that she could help him in these areas, and Marco agreed that he would "give things a go". Marco attended five double therapy sessions, each lasting one-and-a-half hours, and with his mother present for most sessions. However, throughout much of the initial part of the therapy program, Marco was oppositional, although this was interspersed with times of intense engagement in activities. He also often commented that his performance with activities was "not good enough" or "a failure".

Marco understood the concepts with regards to managing his sensory environment well, but he was very reluctant to do any therapy homework between sessions and told the therapist he was able to commit the concepts to memory, which the therapist respected. When discussing the oral sensory system and in particular the four T's of food and drinks that could have a possible regulatory or dysregulatory effect on people (being textures, taste, thickness and temperature), Marco described how his father liked to cook very spicy meals, which often caused disagreements between them as he strongly disliked spicy food. This sparked a discussion on appreciating food differences and possible ways for the family to accommodate each other's likes and dislikes in this area.

Approximately halfway through the therapy process, Marco had an incident at school where he hurt another child and got into trouble with the headteacher. Marco's parents informed the therapist of this with his agreement. When Marco arrived for his next session, he was particularly rude to the therapist at the start. The therapist calmly reminded him about the rule to speak kindly to each other in sessions, told him she was not giving up on him and she could help him develop better self-regulation strategies so that he could have more appropriate behaviour. However, the choice whether to stop or continue with therapy was his and if the latter, Marco's behaviour had to reflect his choice. This meant he had to speak kindly, engage in activities and leave his reading book outside the clinic room – which up to that point he had always taken to sessions and "read" at random times. Marco agreed to the conditions and, from that point on in therapy, made a visible effort to adhere to them.

During the session in which the therapist started addressing problem solving, Marco was easily able to match different types of problems with their corresponding definitions, but he became upset when presented with a range of problem scenarios and when asked to classify them as "easy, hard or complex". However, with encouragement, he persisted and was also able to start identifying some solutions for each with the therapist, including identifying some sensory based strategies that a person could use in the various scenarios if needed to help them regulate better. For example, Marco was able to identify the problem "You are sitting next to a child in class with whom you do not get along. You ask your teacher if you can move to another desk, but he refuses. Your frustration about this is growing daily" as a hard problem. This was because, although the problem was fairly straightforward and had an obvious solution, it was more difficult to solve due to the teacher not agreeing for the child to move to another desk. Some ideas to address this were to ask the teacher to move desks again by explaining the reasons why, or asking a more senior teacher, such as the headteacher, to intervene. In addition, for the child to manage his associated growing frustrations, the child could explore some sensory based activities to help him remain calm until the problem could be resolved.

Further to the above, Marco really enjoyed the role play activities aimed at helping him develop more flexible thinking patterns. One of these related to a situation where a friend did not turn up for a virtual online gaming play date with Marco, which upset him significantly as he thought the friend did it on purpose and did not really want to play with him. The therapist and Marco acted out a scene where they spoke on the phone, first with Marco having the thought "He did not turn up on purpose" in his mind (inflexible thought pattern), and secondly having the thought, "I am not sure why he did not turn up and want to find out" in his mind (flexible thought pattern). Marco was able to immediately identify how the different thought patterns influenced his emotions but also that the conversation where he had a flexible thought pattern played out much more positively than when he had the inflexible thought pattern.

To start addressing Marco's perfectionism, mindset that everything he did was "not good enough" or a "failure" and associated negative self-talk, the therapist discussed famous quotes on perfectionism with him and also encouraged him to be "his own best friend" and speak kindly to himself. The therapist also did the grass head activity with Marco. When discussing the message of this activity, the therapist wrote the words "sunny voice" and "cloudy voice" on two separate cards. She asked Marco to place the "sunny voice" card next to the grass head that grew the most grass, and the "cloudy voice" card next to the one that grew less grass. She then asked him to reverse the cards. This was to explain to Marco that the voice he listened to the most, and which would have the biggest impact on his life, was "in his hands" or within his power to control.

Marco's parents wanted to wait until therapy had concluded before speaking to his teachers about ways to support him, as they felt they wanted to first understand his needs better themselves. Following their meetings with the school, the headteacher requested a meeting with the therapist to better understand Marco's needs and the therapy that was provided. In the meeting with the headteacher, the therapist explained the concepts and some of the strategies that Marco had learnt to help him self-regulate but also the changes that the school could implement to support him considering his complex profile. This included for Marco to be allowed quick movement breaks in class if needed, for the classroom to be aired sufficiently during science/art/food technology lessons, and/or for Marco to be allowed to leave the class for a few minutes when odours became too much for him and for his teachers to allow him the use coloured pens in his book to help him notice text more. In addition, the therapist suggested the headteacher consider providing Marco with the opportunity to meet up with an older pupil with high learning potential who could act as a role model, and/or having a trusted member of staff he could talk to about specific concerns he had in an effort to combat emotionally charged behaviour as a result of feelings that have "built up" over time.

A few months after therapy concluded and also after the new school year had started, Marco's mother reported he was more tolerant to and with others, and they were extremely proud he had not had an anger outburst. She also stated he was more aware and accepting of his sensory hypersensitivities, requesting that his parents reach out to school again to help him with regards to his strong aversion to smells. Marco's parents felt that he still had some way to go with regards to addressing his perfectionism and negative self-talk but stated they had decided to take things at his pace. They stated that what Marco had achieved in occupational therapy was a "great first step", and that they felt more equipped to help him on his journey.

Conclusion

We trust that, having read through the case studies, therapists will now have a better idea and feel more confident in using the DME-C therapy approach's 10 Golden Nuggets and 4 Essential Components to guide their work with children with DME/2e. We truly believe that every therapist has a unique personality, and the authenticity they bring to the therapeutic relationship with a child contributes to successful therapy outcomes; but we also believe that the 10 Golden Nuggets can help therapists further in this quest as it fosters a strengths-based approach to therapy. We also welcome the idea that therapists, as they read through the different case studies and consider how they would have approached each one, may have used completely different activities to achieve the 4 Essential Components of Diarise, Manage transitions, change the Environment and hElp the senses and Communicate.

The DME-C house has a strong foundation and solid walls, but we are excited that therapists, including ourselves, can continually furnish it with known and new activities as we learn and evolve together on our therapeutic journeys.

Notes

* The sport of moving rapidly through an area and negotiating obstacles by running, jumping and climbing but without the aid of equipment. Retrieved and adapted on May 9, 2023. https://en.wikipedia.org/wiki/Parkour.
† An education, health and care plan (EHCP) is a legal document which describes a child or young person's aged up to 25 special educational needs, the support they need, and the outcomes they would like to achieve.
‡ A theraband is a thick, elastic and resistive band normally used for muscle strengthening and/or injury rehabilitation.
§ General Certificate of Secondary Education: A system of public exams taken in various subjects from the age of about 16, or one of these exams, or a qualification from this system. Retrieved from https://dictionary.cambridge.org/dictionary/english/gcse on May 10, 2023.

References

1. Williams, M.S., & Shellenberger, S. (1996). "How Does Your Engine Run?"® A leader's guide to the Alert Program® for self-regulation. Albuquerque, NM: TherapyWorks, Inc.
2. Kuypers, L. (2011) The Zones of Regulation™: A curriculum designed to foster self-regulation and emotional control. Think Social Publishing.
3. Henderson, S.E. and Sugden, D.A. (2007) The Detailed Assessment of Speed of Handwriting. Pearson.

Chapter ten
Resources for Further Help

Introduction

In this chapter, we provide information about organisations that can support occupational therapists to develop their understanding further about children with DME/2e, either generally or when dealing with an individual. Therapists can also signpost families and educators of children with DME/2e to the organisations listed here.

UK-based Organisations

2eMPower

The 2eMPower Project team aims to guide students, parents, teachers, SENDCos and Teaching Assistants (TAs) along a pathway suite of workshops with the strategies and approaches needed to engender confidence, capability and motivation of students with 2e. It was established in 2017 by Professor Sara Rankin of Imperial College London and Dr Susan Smith of GERRIC, University of New South Wales, Sydney, Australia. It is now run by Professor Rankin and her team at Imperial College London.

Contact details

Website: https://www.2empoweruk.org/
Email: 2empower@imperial.ac.uk

British Mensa

British Mensa is a membership society for people of all ages with a high IQ. Although the website does not say anything about including children with DME/2e in their membership, many of its members do have DME/2e.

Contact details

Website: https://mensa.org.uk/
Email: services@mensa.org.uk

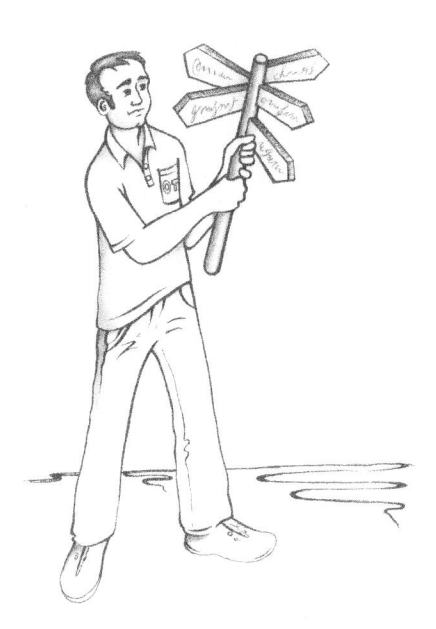

Coram Tomorrow's Achievers

The Tomorrow's Achievers programme provides specialist masterclasses for curious children. The courses are affordable for all and cover a wealth of different topics including science, technology, maths, philosophy, virtual reality, literature and the arts – in ways which involve and challenge the most able students.

Contact details

Website: https://www.tomorrowsachievers.co.uk/
Email: cta@coram.org.uk

The DME Trust

The DME Trust is a partnership between nasen and Potential Plus UK that supports the needs of children with DME/2e. It provides information and advice on DME for children, their families, schools and professionals. They work to advance the understanding of dual or multiple exceptionality and to realise the rights of appropriate education for individuals with DME to help them fulfil their potential.

Contact details

Website: https://potentialplusuk.org/index.php/dme-trust/
Email: info@dmetrust.org

GIFT Courses

GIFT has been supporting the brightest and most curious young minds for 40 years. The organisation runs weekly online Zoom classes, residential weekends, workshop days and Easter and summer schools for secondary age exceptionally able children, including those with DME/2e. These are relaxed, informal opportunities to explore unusual subjects in depth, meet like-minded peers and form lasting friendships.

Contact details

Website: https://www.giftcourses.co.uk/
Email: enquiries@giftcourses.co.uk

nasen (National Association for Special Educational Needs)

nasen is a charitable membership organisation that exists to support and champion those working with, and for, children and young people with SEND and learning differences. The wider nasen family includes The DME Trust (in collaboration with Potential Plus UK) and the Whole School SEND Consortium. There is useful information on these websites about supporting children with DME/2e.

Contact details

Website: https://nasen.org.uk/
Email: welcome@nasen.org.uk

North West Gifted and Talented (NWGT)

NWGT provides support for able learners and their teachers, parents and carers. NWGT works alongside higher education institutions to enrich, extend and challenge the abilities of gifted and talented young people, aiming to improve the attainment, aspirations and motivation of these bright young learners.

Contact details

Website: https://northwestgiftedandtalented.org.uk
Email: aileen.hoare@northwestgiftedandtalented.org.uk

Potential Plus UK

Potential Plus UK is a charity that supports children with HLP, including those with DME/2e. They work to raise awareness about children with HLP and DME/2e and improve the quality of provision and support for them. They also provide a community for young people with HLP and DME/2e and their families. They provide information, advice and guidance services, assessments, training and community activities.

Contact details

Website: https://potentialplusuk.org/
Email: amazingchildren@potentialplusuk.org

The Potential Trust

The Potential Trust provides, promotes and encourages whatever makes education more interesting and exciting for children and young people who have high learning potential or DME/2e by enabling them to access events and experiences that facilitate their personal and social development, their creative, artistic and practical skills as well as their intellectual abilities. They offer bursaries to children with HLP and DME/2e from low and lower income UK-based families to take part in enrichment activities.

Contact details

Website: https://www.thepotentialtrust.org.uk/
Email: thepotentialtrust@clara.co.uk

PowerWood Projects CIC

PowerWood is a UK non-profit dedicated to advocating for and supporting families and individuals living with high-ability neurodiversity in combination with intensity, sensitivity, hyper-reactivity, learning difficulties, uneven development, emotion regulation issues or mental health issues. They celebrate neurodiversity as a natural variation in humans, challenge the social stigmas surrounding being ND and believe that when individuals are given the tools to live fulfilling lives and achieve their aims, neurodiversity is a positive force for change in society. They offer online individual and family support, an online community, blogs and vlogs and an emotional support crisis guide.

Contact details

Website: https://www.powerwood.org.uk
Email: office@powerwood.org.uk

Organisations That Are Accessible from Anywhere

Bright & Quirky

Bright & Quirky is routinely called a "lifeline" for families raising bright kids with learning, social and emotional challenges. They are an online psychoeducation company helping thousands of bright families, with ADHD, anxiety, learning differences like dyslexia and/or those on the autistic spectrum live their happiest, most productive lives. They have a variety of online programs, such as the IdeaLab, the Bright & Quirky Online Summits, the Possibility Plan (a 7 step digital course for parents) and the Video Library.

Contact details

Website: https://brightandquirky.com
Email: support@brightandquirky.com

Gifted and Thriving LLC

Gifted and Thriving is dedicated to the holistic development and support of the gifted/twice-exceptional (2e) community. They have a free 2e Parent Survival Guide and offer services such as family coaching, gifted school programming, workshops, online courses and support groups. Founded by Dr Michael and Julie Postma.

Contact Details

Website: https://www.giftedandthriving.com
Email: support@giftedandthriving.com

The G Word

The G Word is a mosaic of revealing stories told by children, adults and elders that explore giftedness, intelligence and neurodivergent learners across the age spectrum and ask, "In the 21st century, who gets to be gifted and why?" Searching for an answer, The G Word takes an unexpected path, visiting rural, urban and suburban schools, homes of gifted families, low-income neighbourhoods, brain scientists, educators and policy experts to discover that gifted people reside in all walks of life – including even our prisons – but many go unrecognised and don't receive the support they need to fully thrive, sometimes with disastrous consequences. Marc Smolowitz is the director and producer.

Contact details

Website: https://www.thegwordfilm.com
Email: thegwordfilm@gmail.com

The Neurodiversity Podcast

The Neurodiversity Podcast features conversations with neurodivergent people and leaders in the field talking about gifted brains, unusual talents and fresh perspectives. There are many episodes that cover DME/2e. The project has expanded into the Neurodiversity University, where there are professional development and parent online courses about twice exceptionality. Founded by Emily Kircher-Morris.

Contact Details

Website: https://neurodiversitypodcast.com
Email: info@NeurodiversityPodcast.com

Nisai Group (including the Nisai Educational Trust)

Nisai Group provides a virtual academy that has all the positive aspects of a school - the classrooms, qualified teachers, a dedicated support team, extra-curricular activities and form tutors - yet online in an inclusive and secure environment that welcomes every learner. This includes learners with HLP and DME/2e, who can work at their ability rather than age level. Nisai Group has set up the Nisai Educational Trust which has produced some information about children with DME/2e for practitioners working in alternative provision education settings.

Contact details

Website: https://www.nisai.com and https://www.nisai.com/nisaieducationtrust2
Email: info@nisai.com

The OT Company

Children's occupational therapists specialising in working with children with HLP and DME/2e. Online courses for parents on helping children with DME/2e with sensory processing differences cope in real life.

Contact details

Website: https://www.theotcompany.com
Email: mariza@theotcompany.com

TiLT Parenting

TiLT Parenting is an educational resource, podcast, consultancy and community with a focus on positively shifting the way neuro differences in children are perceived, experienced and supported. It was founded in 2016 as a podcast and a community aimed at helping families raising "differently wired" children. Debbie Reber is the founder.

Contact Details

Website: https://tiltparenting.com
Email: info@tiltparenting.com

Organisations in the USA

Belin-Blank Center

The Belin-Blank Center for Gifted Education and Talent Development is a centre at the University of Iowa College of Education. The organisation creates opportunities for equitable talent development. They connect with and provide opportunities for those historically underrepresented in talent development, including children with DME/2e. They provide psychological services and professional learning. They also create original research talent development and connect research to real-world practice. The centre includes an institute of the study of academic acceleration.

Contact Details

Website: https://belinblank.education.uiowa.edu
Email: belinblank@uiowa.edu

Bridges Education Group

The Bridges Education Group includes the Bridges Academy, the Bridges 2e Center, Bridges 2e Media and the Bridges Graduate School of Cognitive Diversity in Education. The group is dedicated to advancing the intellectual, creative and social-emotional lives of students everywhere. They advocate for the development of strength-based and talent-focused educational programmes (SBT) and for further research and development of SBT models, techniques and practices. There are Bridges Academies in Los Angeles and Seattle. There is also an online high school program. The Bridges 2e Center offers programmes for parents of children with DME/2e and an expert advice service.

Contact details

Website: https://bridgeseducationgroup.com
Email: info@bridgeseducationgroup.com

Davidson Institute

Based in Nevada, the mission of the Davidson Institute is to recognise, nurture and support profoundly intelligent young people and to provide opportunities for them to develop their talents to make a positive difference. In order to fulfil this mission, the Davidson Institute offers a free source of resources and general support for families with a profoundly intelligent child, summer programs and online programmes.

Contact details

Website: https://www.davidsongifted.org
Email: info@davidsongifted.org

Gifted Development Center

The Gifted Development Center is based in Colorado. It is the service arm of the Institute of the Study of Advanced Development (ISAD). The Center provides comprehensive assessments and helps parents and families of gifted children understand their legal rights to services within education, plan for the needs of twice-exceptional and highly gifted children and choose the appropriate educational setting.

Contact Details

Website: https://gifteddevelopment.org
Email: gifted@gifteddevelopment.com

Gifted Homeschoolers Forum (GHF)

GHF's mission is to empower every gifted family to make strategic, proactive and intentional educational choices. It is a supportive community for gifted learners, including those with DME/2e, and their families. They provide connections that bring the children and their families together and information that helps support them to lead happy and healthy lives.

Contact Details

Website: https://ghflearners.org
Twitter: www.twitter.com/ghflearners

National Association for Gifted Children (NAGC)

Based in the USA, NAGC is a membership organisation that aims to empower all who support children with advanced abilities in accessing equitable opportunities that develop their gifts and talents. They do this through advocacy, outreach, education and research.

Contact Details

Website: https://nagc.org
Email: nagc@nagc.org

REEL2e

REEL2e strives to ensure Silicon Valley's twice-exceptional students thrive in school by raising parent and educator awareness and understanding of practical, research-based strategies to address their needs successfully. For educators, they create and curate resources, workshops and programs to help them make school a place where learners with DME/2e can be successful. For parents, they organise and disseminate events and tools to help parents learn to advocate for and support their 2e kids.

Contact details

Website: https://www.reel2e.org
Email: hello@reel2e.org

Smart Kids with Learning Disabilities

Smart Kids with Learning Disabilities provides information, support and inspiration to parents of children with learning disabilities and attention deficit disorders, while also educating the public about the remarkable gifts and talents of these kids. There is a website and blog, free newsletter and regional educational programs which empower parents to become effective advocates for their children. Smart Kids also emphasises the importance of nurturing a child's interests and strengths and works to dispel the stigma and misconceptions about learning disabilities and attention deficit disorders.

Contact details

Website: https://www.smartkidswithld.org
Email: info@smartkidswithld.org

Summit Center

Summit Center provides educational and psychological assessments, consultations and counselling services for children, their parents and families. They work with all kids – including those who are gifted, those with learning challenges and those who are both gifted and have challenges. Summit Center has assembled an expert team of professionals and specialists, who are dedicated to using a strengths-based approach to help children reach their fullest developmental potential. They are based in California.

Contact Details

Website: https://summitcenter.us
Email: inquiry@summitcenter.us

Supporting Emotional Needs of the Gifted (SENG)

SENG is a USA-based nonprofit organisation that empowers families and communities to guide gifted and talented individuals to reach their goals intellectually, physically, emotionally, socially and spiritually. SENG provides support through a variety of programs, including online support groups for gifted, talented and twice-exceptional individuals and their parents/guardians, online SENGinars with leading experts, in-person regional mini-conferences and an annual conference, SENG Model Parent Groups (SMPG) and Facilitator Training, SENG Library, SENGVine e-newsletter, Continuing Education courses for professionals, workshops and more.

Contact Details

Website: https://www.sengifted.org
Email: office@sengifted.org

Twice Exceptional Children's Advocacy (TECA)

Twice Exceptional Children's Advocacy's mission is to help parents understand what twice exceptionality is and help them identify whether their children are 2e. They assist parents in finding and advocating for the education and resources their children require. TECA provides parents with a one-stop source for 2e, so they can spend less time searching for information and resources and more time with their child and family. They also offer support groups and community online forums for parents of 2e children.

Contact Details

Website: https://www.teca2e.org
Email: info@teca2e.org

With Understanding Comes Calm LLC

With Understanding Comes Calm is a USA-based company that provides guidance for parents of children with DME/2e as well as educator training and mentoring for adults. The organisation also provides Let's Talk 2e parent, educator and DME/2e adult conferences. Julie Skolnik is the founder.

Contact Details

Website: https://www.withunderstandingcomescalm.com
Email: julie@withunderstandingcomescalm.com

210 Resources for Further Help

Organisations in Australasia

Australian Association for the Education of the Gifted and Talented (AAEGT)

The Australian Association for the Education of the Gifted and Talented is a national organisation committed to furthering the education and wellbeing of gifted students. It is a not-for-profit company. Through evidence-based leadership, advocacy, collaboration, education and communication, the AAEGT strives for the vision that all gifted students across the nation are recognised and have their intellectual and affective needs met through appropriate educational provision. There are regional websites, and the organisation runs an annual Gifted Awareness Week.

Contact Details

Website: https://www.aaegt.net.au
Email: info@aaegt.net.au

Australian Gifted Support Centre (AGSC)

Based in Sydney, the Australian Gifted Support Centre has a team of qualified educators and counsellors who specialise in supporting gifted children, including those with a learning difficulty such as dyslexia and conditions such as ADHD and autism. They offer assessments and a wide range of services to assist families with bright children, including resources and courses.

Contact Details

Website: https://australiangiftedsupport.com
Email: enquiries@australiangiftedsupport.com

Gifted 2e Support

Gifted 2e Support is an Australian registered business providing services for people with twice exceptionality (2e), their families and others who support them. While they have some paid staff, they are primarily run by volunteers. Their focus is consultancy, advocacy and support for parents, families and those that work with twice exceptionality (2e), neurodiverse and gifted people Australia-wide. Founded by Amanda Drury.

Contact Details

Website: https://gifted2esupport.com.au
Email: admin@gifted2esupport.com.au

Kids Like Us (KLU)

Kids Like Us is an Australia-based company that provides support for young people with 2e, their parents and professionals with parental, learning, and daily living strategies, contacts, advocacy and products which may assist twice-exceptional people to succeed and become the great adults they have the potential to be. KLU offers counselling and psychology services, teaching and tutoring, social and emotional support groups, peer support, advocacy and parent support.

Contact Details

Website: https://kidslikeus.org.au

Our Gifted Kids

Our Gifted Kids is an Australia-based hub for all things gifted. They bring parents, professionals and businesses together as a community to talk and support each other, making everyone's lives easier. There is a podcast, a community for kids, online courses for parents and a blog. Founded by Sophia Elliott.

Contact Details

Website: https://ourgiftedkids.com

New Zealand Association for Gifted Children (NZAGC)

NZAGC is a charitable organisation that supports gifted children, including those with DME/2e, and their families. They publish *Tall Poppies* magazine, lobby government and educational circles, organise national workshops for teachers, parents and children and assist parents to set up local branches.

Contact Details

Website: https://www.giftedchildren.org.nz
Email: info@giftedchildren.org.nz

Glossary

Adaptations (minor and major)   In the context of occupational therapy provision for children with sensory impairments and complex physical needs, adaptations are the physical changes brought about to a child's home, school and/or other relevant environments to enable them to access it. An example of a minor adaptation is a stair handrail, and a major adaptation is a through floor wheelchair lift.

ADHD (attention deficit hyperactivity disorder)   A lifelong neurodevelopmental disorder characterised by a persistent pattern of inattention and/or hyperactivity and impulsivity, which makes focussing on everyday requests and routines challenging, affecting all areas of a person's functioning.

Alternative provision (AP)   Places that provide full-time education for children who cannot go to a mainstream school because of exclusion, illness or other reasons.

ASD/ASC (autism spectrum disorder/autism spectrum condition/autism/autistic)   A lifelong neurodevelopmental condition characterised by different communication styles and preferences and persistent difficulties with neurotypical social communication and interaction. Autistic people often display stereotypical behaviour, experience sensory processing differences, have highly focussed and/or restricted interests or hobbies, are resistant to change and can experience intense anxiety.

Assistive technology   In the context of occupational therapy provision for children with sensory impairments and complex physical needs, assistive technology is the umbrella term for devices, equipment and software used to enable children to live more independently.

Asynchronous development   Refers to uneven intellectual, academic, physical and emotional development. In typically developing children, these aspects of development progress at about the same rate. That is, the development is in "sync". However, in children with high learning potential and DME/2e, these areas of development develop unevenly or are out of "sync".

Auditory sensory system   The sensory system in the human body responsible for perceiving sounds from the environment.

Avoiding/avoider   See "sensory over responsive".

Blended education   Blended education, also known as hybrid education, is an approach to education that combines online educational materials and opportunities for interaction online with traditional place-based classroom learning.

CAMHS (child and adolescent mental health services)   Statutory services that support children and young people with their mental health.

Dabrowski's overexcitabilities   The Polish psychologist Kazimierz Dabrowski identified five areas in which children with high learning potential exhibit intense behaviours, also known as "overexcitabilities" or "hypersensitivities": psychomotor, sensual, emotional, intellectual and imaginational.

DCD (developmental coordination disorder) A lifelong neurodevelopmental motor skills disorder that affects a person's fine and/or gross motor coordination and cannot be explained by physical, sensory or intellectual impairments. In some countries, the term "dyspraxia" is used as a substitute for DCD or interchangeably with DCD.

DME (dual or multiple exceptionality) A term used to describe individuals with high learning potential who also have a special educational need or disability.

DME-C therapy approach or DME-C approach The therapy approach or practical guide created to support occupational therapists to help children with HLP and DME/2e who have challenges specifically relating to sensory processing, unhelpful thought patterns and self-regulation. It also contains guidance on how therapists can approach therapy when addressing other challenges children with HLP and DME/2e may face that impact on their occupational performance.

Dyscalculia A specific and persistent difficulty in understanding numbers that can lead to a range of maths related difficulties.

Dysgraphia Handwriting difficulties.

Dyslexia A specific learning difficulty that primarily affects the skills involved in accurate and fluent word reading and spelling, characterised by difficulties in phonological awareness, verbal memory and verbal processing speed.

Dyspraxia The difficulty to plan, organise and carry out a sequence of unfamiliar actions and to do what one needs to do or wants to do, forming part of DCD. However, dyspraxia is also classified under the umbrella term of Dr Lucy Miller's Sensory Processing Disorder Model, subtype sensory based motor disorder.

Educational psychologist A psychologist concerned with a child's learning and development, who uses specialist skills in psychology and educational assessment techniques to help children who have difficulties in learning, behaviour and social adjustment.

EHCP (education and health care plan, or EHC plan) A legal document that describes a child's special educational needs or disabilities, the support they need and the outcomes they would like to achieve.

Emotional control, emotional regulation, emotional self-regulation See "self-regulation".

Exclusion (in a school context) A term used in the UK for when a child is excluded from school on a temporary (also called suspension) or permanent basis for breaching the school's behaviour policy.

Executive functioning A set of processes that all have to do with managing oneself and one's resources in order to achieve a goal.

Fixed mindset Having the belief that intelligence is fixed, and that intellectual abilities cannot be developed.

Flexible thinking Having or possessing different ways of perceiving the motives and intents of others and difficult or problematic situations.

Gustatory sensory system The sensory system in the human body responsible for perceiving taste.

Gifted and talented (G&T) A term used to describe children who have high learning potential in an education context. The term was used in England for the government's gifted and talented strategy between 1997 and 2011.

Gifted See "high learning potential".
Growth mindset Having the belief that intelligence can be developed through hard work and that an individual can "grow their brain" by focussing on the process which leads to learning.
Hearing impairment When a person is unable to hear as well as someone with normal hearing, with the impairment ranging from mild to severe and affecting one or both ears.
Helpful thought patterns The umbrella term used for the common types of thought patterns that help a child to feel regulated and "up to doing a task". It includes positive self-talk, flexible thinking and the ability to define or categorise problems in order to solve them.
High learning potential (HLP) A term used to describe children who are endowed with an unusual natural ability, intelligence or talent. It is a term used instead of "gifted" in the UK.
Hypersensitivity See "sensory over responsive".
Inflexible thinking Having or possessing only one way of viewing the motives and intents of others and difficult or problematic situations.
Instant explosion A term developed as part of the DME-C therapy approach to refer to a child with DME/2e who, due to a variety of reasons, may harbour a distrust of authority figures. When engaging in occupational therapy, the child shows their true feelings from the start by being very vocal and openly resistant.
Intellectual boredom When a child with DME/2e is not challenged adequately on a cognitive level and subsequently feels bored. This often leads to challenging and unacceptable behaviour.
Learning difference A condition that creates an obstacle to a specific form of learning for a person, but which does not affect their overall IQ.
Learning difficulty See "learning difference".
Learning disability A condition that affects a person's learning and intelligence across all areas of their life.
Interoception Sensing the basic functions or physical conditions of the body, such as hunger or thirst, and involved in emotional regulation.
More able or most able Terminology used since 2012 to identify children who are achieving highly in education in England.
Negative self-talk Self-talk that is negative in nature, also referred to as a "pessimistic or cloudy voice". It makes it hard for a child to feel regulated and "up to doing a task", whatever that task may be.
Negative thought patterns The thought patterns concerned with a person being critical of themselves and negative self-talk.
Neurodivergent A term used to describe individuals whose brains process, learn or behave differently from what we may consider "typical". It may be used by those with formal diagnoses such as dyslexia, ADHD or those on the autistic spectrum to describe themselves and their needs. It may also be used by those without a formal diagnosis, but who experience behaviours and traits that impact their daily lives, meaning that they identify as being part of the wider neurodiverse community.

Neurodiverse/neurodiversity This refers to a community that includes, accepts and celebrates the diversity in human brain function and cognition resulting in different ways of thinking, processing and learning.

Neurotypical Describes a way of thinking, perceiving and behaving in ways that are considered the norm by the general population.

nasen The short-hand name used by the National Association for Special Educational Needs in the UK.

Non-OT factors An umbrella term developed as part of the DME-C therapy approach to refer to some of the common characteristics that children with HLP across the world share as reported by their parents, including asynchronous development and social isolation, that can cause children with HLP and DME/2e to have social, emotional, mental health and behavioural difficulties (root causes) and/or can impact on occupational therapy. As the common characteristics can also positively impact on occupational therapy, **all** of the common characteristics are included in the term "non-OT factors".

OCD (obsessive compulsive disorder) A mental health condition where the individual has obsessions which are unwanted, intrusive thoughts and images that causes distress and compulsions which are the behaviours the individual engages in to try and get rid of the obsessions in order to decrease their distress.

Olfactory sensory system The sensory system in the human body responsible for perceiving smells/odours.

Oral sensory system see "gustatory sensory system"

OT (occupational therapy or occupational therapist) A client-centred health profession concerned with promoting health and wellbeing through occupation. The primary goal of occupational therapy is to enable people to participate in the activities of everyday life. Occupational therapists achieve this outcome by working with people and communities to enhance their ability to engage in the occupations they want to, need to, are expected to do or by modifying the occupation or the environment to better support their occupational engagement (WFOT, 2012).

OT-factors An umbrella term developed as part of the DME-C therapy approach to refer to the sensory or motor skills deficits and challenges, and associated difficulties with emotional self-regulation, that can cause children with HLP and DME/2e to have social, emotional, mental health and behavioural difficulties (root causes).

Paediatric The healthcare branch of medicine and therapy provision for children aged 0 – 25.

PDA (pathological demand avoidance) A profile on the autism spectrum involving resisting and avoiding everyday demands and a need for control driven by anxiety, which has a significant impact on an individual's everyday life and wellbeing.

Play dough thinking See "flexible thinking".

Positive self-talk Self-talk that is positive in nature, also referred to as an "optimistic or sunny voice". It helps a child to feel regulated and "up to doing a task", whatever that task may be.

Processing speed The amount of time it takes to perceive and process information and formulate or enact a response.

Proprioceptive sensory system   The sensory system in the human body responsible for perceiving body position and muscle control.

Psychiatrist   A medical doctor who specialises in mental health, concerned with the diagnosis, treatment (including prescribing medication) and prevention of mental health conditions.

Registration/bystander   See "sensory under responsive".

School refusal   A term used in the UK to describe a regular refusal to attend school or routine problems staying at school. Children may avoid school to cope with stress or fear for a vast number of reasons.

Self-regulation   The ability of a person to independently monitor if they feel calm, ready or "up to the task" for the various activities they engage in throughout the day. In other words, whether a person can appropriately meet the occupational and/or self-regulatory demands of that particular activity and to adjust as necessary. The ability to appropriately self-regulate develops throughout childhood. Difficulties with self-regulation can be due to a variety of reasons such as sensory processing differences, unhelpful thought patterns, attention difficulties, anxiety and emotional distress, to name but a few.

SEND (special educational needs or disabilities)   The term used in England to describe children or young people who have a learning difficulty or disability which calls for special educational provision to be made for him or her.

SENDCO/SENCO (special educational needs and disabilities coordinator)   In England, the SENDCO, who must be a qualified teacher, oversees the strategic development of SEND policy and provision and ensures the implementation of the SEND policy on a day-to-day basis.

Seeking/seeker   See "sensory seeking".

Self-talk   A type of thought pattern, the way a person talks to themself, or a person's "inner voice".

Sensitivity/sensor   See "sensory over responsive".

Sensory diet   An individualised plan of sensory based activities which is scheduled into a child's day to address their sensory processing differences.

Sensory environment   Developed as part of the DME-C therapy approach, "sensory environment" is the umbrella term for a child's sensory processing differences that impact on their modulation, self-regulation and activity participation (their feelings and behaviours). Addressing a child's sensory environment in therapy means addressing the child's sensory processing differences, including the sensual and/or psychomotor overexcitabilities that impact on them.

Sensory impairment   The common term to describe visual impairment, blindness, hearing impairment, deafness and deafblindness.

Sensory processing difficulties or differences   Difficulties with sensory integration. In other words, when the brain has difficulty registering, interpreting and organising sensory messages received through the senses from the environment and/or from within the body, resulting in inappropriate motor and/or behavioural responses, meaning that the child struggles to successfully interact with their environment.

SPD or sensory processing disorder, sensory regulation dysfunction, sensory integration dysfunction, sensory dysfunction disorder See "sensory processing difficulties or differences".

Speech and language impairment or delay When speech and language is severely behind the typical population and does not follow the expected pattern of development, or when speech and language develop in the normal pattern of development but at a slower rate.

Speech and language therapist A healthcare professional who provides treatment, support and care for children and adults who have difficulties with communication and/or with eating, drinking and swallowing.

Speech pathologist, speech and language pathologist See "speech and language therapist".

SI (sensory integration) The neurological process by which the brain registers, interprets and organises sensory messages received through the senses from the environment and/or from within the body in order to have appropriate motor and/or behavioural responses so a person can successfully interact with their environment.

Sensory seeking When a child noticeably seeks out more of a particular sensation or sensory stimulus than those around them, but in doing so can get over stimulated and may not become calmer and more regulated.

Sensory over responsive When a child is more sensitive to a particular sensation or sensory stimulus than other people, perceiving a "normal" sensation as harmful, resulting in the child having a "fight, flight or freeze response".

Sensory under responsive When a child is less aware of a particular sensation or sensory stimulus than other people and needs more or a higher intensity of the stimulus before they will respond.

Slow burner A term developed as part of the DME-C therapy approach to refer to a child with DME/2e who, due to a variety of reasons, may harbour a distrust of authority figures. When engaging in occupational therapy, the child may try to hide their true feelings, with resistance to participating in therapy sessions and engaging with therapy homework between sessions, increasing over time.

Social, emotional, mental health issues and behavioural difficulties A type of SEND where children and young people have severe difficulties in managing their emotions and behaviour, often showing inappropriate responses to feelings and situations.

Social isolation The lack of social contact with peers and/or having no or few like minded friends to interact with regularly.

Solid thinking See "inflexible thinking".

Statutory services A type of government mandated care or service to the public in the UK. Examples are child support and health care, including assessment services.

S-TE-DD-R Developed as part of the DME-C therapy approach's essential component 3 "change the Environment and hElp the senses", the S-TE-DD-R guidelines refer to a systematic way for therapists to address a child's sensory and thought environments. The acronym was chosen for its similarity to the word "steadier" in sound, with the letters representing the words subdivide, teach and experience/explore, discuss and discover and remember.

Tactile sensory system   The sensory system in the human body responsible for perceiving touch.

Thought environment   Developed as part of the DME-C therapy approach, "thought environment" is the umbrella term for the thought patterns that impact on a child's modulation, self-regulation and activity participation (their feelings and behaviours). Addressing a child's thought environment in therapy means addressing the child's unhelpful thought patterns including the emotional, imaginational and, to an extent, the intellectual overexcitabilities that impact on them.

Transition or transitions   To change or move from one activity, environment, state, subject or situation to another.

Twice exceptional (2e)   See "DME/dual or multiple exceptionality."

Unhelpful thought patterns   The umbrella term used for the common types of thought patterns that make it hard for a child to feel regulated and "up to doing a task". It includes perfectionism, negative self-talk, inflexible thinking and preoccupation with problems that affect a child's activity participation.

Vestibular sensory system   The sensory system in the human body responsible for perceiving movement and balance.

Visual impairment   A loss of sight that cannot be corrected by glasses or contact lenses, affecting one or both eyes.

Visual sensory system   The sensory system in the human body responsible for perceiving visual images from the environment.

Working memory   One of the brain's executive functions; a skill that allows people to work with information without losing track of what they are doing. Remembering a phone number, recalling directions or performing calculations are all tasks that use working memory.

INDEX

2e *see* dual or multiple exceptionality

acute social awareness 54, 64
ADHD 61, 77-82, 175-80, 184; definition 77; executive functioning 80; impulsivity 78, 81; low self-esteem 80, 81; misdiagnosis 79; recommended therapy approach 81-3; session length 107; social and emotional development 80
Alert Programme 153
alternative provision 25, 205
anxiety: cause examples 122, 131-2; cause of explosive behaviour 162; dual or multiple exceptionality characteristics 45; high learning potential characteristics 19, 24, 32, 34, 36; important of positive relationships 56; in ADHD 81; in autism 70, 71-72; in case studies 173, 175, 178, 179, 180, 181; in PDA 137; in sensory processing differences 87; prevalence in high learning potential 33; reducing transition-related 136, 138; transitions 135, 161
arguing 17, 108, 110, 132, 133, 175, 182
Asperger's Disorder 70, 73, **74-75**
assessment: ADHD 79; autism 73; dual or multiple exceptionality 156; of strengths and needs 67
assistive technology 62
asynchronous development 27-31, *28*, 35; being mindful of 141; effect on social and emotional development 31, 66; examples 30-31, 111-2, 158, 173, 187; in ADHD 79; in dual or multiple exceptionality 40-41, 44, 45, 56; need for occupational therapy 63
attention deficit hyperactivity disorder *see* ADHD
auditory sensitivity: examples 121-2, 134, 168, 170, 171, 173, 181, 184, 190; example using S-TE-DD-R **144**; high learning potential with sensory processing differences 93; report writing 157, 159; Sensory Discrimination Disorder 97; Sensory Modulation Disorder 91; sensory trigger 131, 133; session summary *146*
auditory sensory system 88, 97, **144**, 160
autism 61, 65, 70-8, 86, 192; common difficulties 70-2; communication difficulties 70, 71; definition 70-1;

misdiagnosis 72-3; recommended therapy approach 77-8
Autism Level Up! 153
autism spectrum disorder/condition *see* autism
avoiding/avoider *see* over responsiveness
Ayres Sensory Integration (ASI) 70
Ayres, Anna Jean 85

backward chaining 77
blended provision 25
boredom 23, 24, **32**, 45, 63, 64-5; ADHD 79, 82; analysing emotional state 153; example 65; in case studies 177, 191; increased sensory seeking behaviour 96; reviewing diary 133; with repetition 112-3
boundaries *104*, 107-10, *165*
building relationships 108, 110; with peers 56
bullying 35

CAMHS 62-63
cerebral palsy 61
challenging behaviour 36, 64, 110, 113
change the Environment (Essential Component) 129, 139-50, 154
Characteristics of Giftedness Scale 15-6
Child and Adolescent Mental Health Service *see* CAMHS
cipher activities 114-6
Cognitive Orientation to Daily Occupational Performance 70, 77, 120, 188, 193
Columbus Group 27
common language 152, 153-4, *166*
Communicate (Essential Component) 129, 152-4
communication 109; advocacy 102; behaviour as 36; development of 88; to support dual or multiple exceptional children 56, 67; with children 109, 110-2, 113;
compassion 15, 18-9, **32**, 150, 177
concentration **74**, 81, 87, 106, 132, 157, 159; in case studies 173, 175, 176, 178
CO-OP Approach *see* Cognitive Orientation to Daily Occupational Performance
coping strategies 113-4
creativity 108; of child 108; of therapist 121
curiosity: dual or multiple exceptional characteristics 44, **46**; high learning

potential characteristics 14, 15, 17-8, 22, **32**; in case studies 180, 186, 191; in therapy 112, 139, 150, 151

Dabrowski, Kazimierz 32-3
Dabrowski's Overexcitabilities *see* overexcitabilties
DASH 69
DCD 61, 63, 68-70, 97, 131; auditory attention 69; auditory memory 69; executive functioning 69; in case studies 171, 187, 190; in reports 157, 158; recommended therapy approach 70, 98; visio-spatial functioning 69
delayed outcomes 116-9, 147
depression 24, 33, 36, 45, 80, 87, 162
Detailed Assessment of Speed of Handwriting *see* DASH
developmental coordination disorder *see* DCD
Diarise (Essential Component) 129-35, 154; in case studies 168, 182, 185, 191
direct language *104*, 110-2, 113, *165*
Discuss & Discover (S-TE-DD-R) 140, 141
disengagement from education 36, 45, 52, 65, 113
Diagnostic and Statistical Manual of Mental Disorders, Fifth Edition *see* DSM-V
disorganisation **23**, 26, *46*, *48*, 49, *50*, 54, 68; in case studies 180, 190, 192
distraction **143**, 167, 184, 196
distrust of authority 66, 108-9
DME Trust 6, 52, 56, 201
DME *see* dual or multiple exceptionality
DME-C therapy approach 67, 77, 82, 99, 100, 103; effectiveness 6-9
DSM-V 68, 72, 78, 87, 100
dual or multiple exceptionality: assessment 156; barriers 51-3; characteristics 44-9, **46**, *47*, *49*; definition 1, 39, 61; describing in reports 157-9; difficulties 49-51; examples 40-1; famous people 58-9; frequency in population 42; needs 45-6, **46**; portrayal in the media 57-8; scenarios 53-4; strengths 45-6, **46**; support needed 54-7; identification 42
Dunn, Winnie 85, 90
Dweck, Carol 123-4
dyscalculia 61
dysgraphia *see* handwriting difficulties
dyslexia 61, 170
dyspraxia 68-70, 96-7; recommended therapy approach 98
dysregulation **23**, 112, 118, 126, 131, 134, 135, 145, 154; in case studies 168, 178, 183, 185, 197

echolalia 71
Education Health Care Plan (EHCP) 52
Ehlers-Danlos Syndrome (EDS) 69
Einstein, Albert 59, 77, 78, **149**
emotional outbursts: as a form of communication 36; as a reason for seeking therapy 117, 131; as part of At-Risk Profile 25; as part of emotional overexcitability 34; caused by emotional sensitivity 21, 24; caused by inflexible thinking **148**; caused by perfectionism 36, 45, **147**, 158; in case studies 168, 169, 172-5, 175-7, 188, 195; in examples *50*, 111-2, 135, 158; out of context to the situation **150**
emotional overexcitability 32, 34, 94, 110
emotional regulation *see* self-regulation
emotional sensitivity 18, 21-2, 24, 45, 94, 108, 177
empathy 25, **32**, 55, 64, **75**
Essential Components 3-4, 114, 129-55, 164, *166*
executive functioning 44, 47, 49, 51; in ADHD 80; in DCD 69

Falck, Sonja 53, 56-7
fear of failure *46*, *47*, *48*, *50*, 64, 107, 116, 117, **147**, 161, 195
fine motor skills 28, *43*, 64, 69, 110, 118; in case studies 176, 193
fixed mindset 23, 64, 82, 116, 123-5
flexible thinking **148**, 151, 161; in case studies 169, 174, 182, 185, 197
friendships 71, 78, 80, 81, 87, 111; in case studies 172, 180, 187, 195
frustration: as a cause of behavioural issues 36, 109, 158; as a cause of poor mental health 36; as part of dual or multiple exceptional profile 26, 29, 39, *46*, *47*, *48*, *50*; caused by asynchronous development 28, 29, *43*, 44; in case studies 180, 193, 194, 197; in therapy 106; perfectionism 19, 36, 159

Gifted Development Center 31, 207
giftedness *see* high learning potential
Giftedness/Asperger's Disorder Checklist (GADC) 73-6
goal setting 51, 67, 70, 159-61; examples 160-1
Golden Nuggets 3-4, 67, 99, 150, 164, *165*
grass heads activity 118, 147, 151
gross motor skills 28, 69, 120
growth mindset *104*, 123-5, *165*
gustatory sensory system 88, 94, 97, 160, 191, 195, 197

handwriting difficulties 52, 61, 69, 76, 120, 133, 176
handwriting speed 69, 76
hearing impairment *see* sensory impairments
heavy work *see* proprioception
hElp the senses (Essential Component) 129, 139-50, 154
high learning potential (HLP) 11-37; and ADHD 78-82; and autism 72-7; and DCD 68-70; characteristics 15-22, 35, 63-4, 121, 141, 150; definition 11-3, 27; frequency in population 15; identification 14-5, 65
High Learning Potential/Autism/DME (HADC) Checklist **73-6**
HLP *see* high learning potential
home education 25, 52, 170, 183, 189
hyperactivity 45, 78
hyperfocus 79
hypersensitivity *see* overexcitability

ICD-11 68, 72, 78, 100
imaginational overexcitability 32, 34-5, 79, 94, 120, 135
imposter syndrome 102-3
impulsivity 23, 45
inattentiveness 78
Incredible 5-Point Scale 153
inflexible thinking **148**, 150, 161; in case studies 168, 177, 182, 185, 190, 192, 196, 198
intellectual overexcitability **32**, 34, 94, 106, 139
International Classification of Diseases and Related Health Problems *see* ICD-11
interoception 90
isolation 25, 45, 63, 66

justice, sense of 20-1, 64, 134, 147, 148, 154, 175, 177

MABC-2 *see* Movement ABC-2
Mackie, Susan 124
Manage transitions (Essential Component) 129, 135-9, 154
Mandich, Angela 70
Mensa 102, 156, 200
mental health difficulties 36, 45, 52, 61, 63
Miller, Lucy 90
Mind Ninja 153
Mindfulmazing 153
misunderstanding: about high learning potential 28, 29, 35, 36; about dual or multiple exceptionality 51, 52, 63, 81; about the term gifted 12; between parent and child 105-6; in case studies 178

Model of Sensory Processing 85, 90, 92, 93
modelling: growth mindset 125-6; common language 153, 154; communication 152
monitoring one's responses 110-2
Moro reflex 171, 187
motor coordination difficulty 157, 158, 180
motor skills deficits 63, 77
Movement ABC-2 158
multi exceptionality *see* dual or multiple exceptionality
muscular dystrophy 61

naming feelings 132, 152
nasen 42, 202
negative thought patterns: in case studies 164, 169; hindering participation 131; strategies to address 116, 117, 118, 121, 129; 146, **147-9**, 151
neurodivergence 12, 100
neurological differences 61, 67
neurological thresholds 92, *92*
non-OT factors 63-7, 69, 77, 82
noughts and crosses activity 143

obsessive compulsive disorder (OCD) *41*, 58, 59, 181
OEs *see* overexcitabilities
OEQ-II *see* Overexcitability Questionnaire-Two
olfactory sensitivity 143-4, 195
olfactory sensory system 88, **143**, 195
oral sensitivity 143, 177
oral sensory system *see* gustatory sensory system
overexcitabilities 31-36, **32**, 79, 82, 85, 93, 141
Overexcitability Questionnaire-Two 33
overlearning 112-4
over-responsiveness 71, *92*, *93*, 94, 95, 133, 159

Pathological Demand Avoidance *see* PDA
PDA 137
perfectionism: characteristic of dual or multiple exceptionality 45, 47, *50*, 64, 107; characteristic of high learning potential 15, 19, 36; in case studies 168, 173, 180-1, 187, 190, 192-5, 197-8; in examples 158, 159, 161; non-OT factors 77, 82, 111; strategies to address 116, 117, **147**, 161
Pfeiffer, Steven 12-3
physical disabilities 61-2
Piechowski, Michael 33
Polatajko, Helene J.Positive Disintegration, Theory of 32-3

postural disorder 96; recommended therapy approach 98
Potential Plus UK 4, 6, 12, 13, 31, 45, 102, 156, 203
Potential Trust, The 5, 203
practical activities 114-6
praise 23, 56, 124
problem classification system 148-9, 168, 174-5, 185-6, 194, 197
processing speed 23, 40, 43, *43*, 49-51, 184
Profiles of the Gifted and Talented 22-7
proprioception: activities **142**, 146; example of sensory discrimination difficulty 97, in case studies 179, 190, 191, 193; in psychomotor overexcitability 96; in therapy sessions 160; sensory system 89-90,
psychomotor overexcitability 32, 33, 79, 82, 93, 94, 95

questioning authority 24, 64, 66

referral: to another professional 8, 67, 73, 77-8, 131, 162
registration/bystander *see* under responsiveness
Remember (S-TE-DD-R) 142
repetition *see* overlearning
right and wrong, sense of *see* justice, sense of
Ronksley-Pavia's Model of Twice Exceptionality 41

salad spinner paintings 117, 147
seeking/seeker *see* sensory seeking
self-awareness 63, 131, 135, 141
self-regulation: activities to develop skills 110, 115, 129, 139, 141, **144**, 154; and growth mindset 125; assessment of 156, 157, 159; difficulties as a characteristic of asynchronous development 28, *28*; difficulties as a characteristic of dual or multiple exceptionality 44, 45, 47, 49, 51; in case studies 175, 177, 184, 186, 197; in therapy 63, 103, 106, 153, 160-1; sensory 90, 92
self-talk: activities to address negative 118, **147-8**, 150-1; in case studies 167, 169, 182, 185, 192, 198; in imposter syndrome 103; in therapy *151*, 161
SEND *see* special educational need or disability
sense of belonging 66-7
sense of self 25, 108
sensory based motor disorders 68, 91, 96-7; recommended therapy approach 98
sensory diet 81, 82, 83
sensory discrimination disorder 91, 97

sensory dysfunction disorder *see* sensory processing differences
sensory environment 132, 140-1, 142-4
sensory impairments 61-2
sensory integration 85
sensory integration dysfunction *see* sensory processing differences
Sensory Ladders 153
sensory modulation 77, 141
sensory modulation disorder 90-93; recommended therapy approach 98
sensory over responsiveness *see* over responsiveness
sensory processing differences: ADHD 79, 81, 82; assessment 157-9; autism 72, 77; definition 85; dual or multiple exceptionality 44, 47, 49, 61, 86-91; high learning potential 21, 93; in case studies 167, 173, 180, 183, 187, 190, 193, 195-6; informing parents 106; overexcitabilities 33, 93-6, *95*; prevalence 93; therapy approach 98, 129-55; therapy method 103-26; therapy to support 63
sensory processing difficulties *see* sensory processing differences
sensory processing disorder 68, 100
Sensory Processing Disorder Model 85, 90, 91, *93*
sensory processing patterns 77, 90, 92
sensory regulation dysfunction *see* sensory processing differences
sensory seeking *92*, *93*, 94, *95*; in case studies 167, 181, 184, 190, 195, 197
sensory sensitivity 21-2; in autism 70
sensory systems 87, *88-90*
sensory under responsiveness *see* under responsiveness
sensual overexcitability 32-3, **32**; example 34; hypersensitivity 35; ADHD 79; sensory processing and 93-4, *95*, 139
session length 106-7
session summary sheet 146, 151; example 146, 151
Silverman, Linda 15, 31
SPD *see* sensory processing disorder
special educational need or disability 1, 29, 39, 61
speech and language delay 61-2
spiky profile 66
S-TE-DD-R 140-5
Subdivide (S-TE-DD-R) 141
Super WOW factor 121-3

tactile defensiveness 63, 109, 134, 142, 154, 173, 195
tactile sensitivity 171, 187

tactile sensory system 88, 97, 160, 171, 173, 195
Teach & Experience/Explore (S-TE-DD-ER) 141
therapy: contract 82; discontinuing 162, 189; goals 67; homework 66, 114, 120, 146, 147, 151
thought environment: addressing 146, **147-50**, *151*, 160, 162, *166*; developing awareness of 139, 140-1, 154; in case studies 181, 185, 188, 189, 191, 193; triggers for feelings and behaviour 131
TPD *see* Positive Disintegration, Theory of
Trail, Beverly 56
trauma 131
triggers 131-5, 152, 154, 167, 168
Tripartite Model of Giftedness 12-3
twice exceptionality *see* dual or multiple exceptionality

underachievement 36, 54, 56-7, 80
under responsiveness 70, 92, *92*, 93, *93*, 157, 173, 176, 196

unexpected outcomes 116-9, 146
unhelpful thought patterns: activities to address 115, 121, 123, 125; in case studies 170, 174, 176, 179, 181, 194; therapy approach 129, 131, 141, 150, *151*, 166; therapy method 103, 113

vestibular sensory system *89*, 91, 96, 139, **142**, 159, 160
visual impairment *see* sensory impairments
visual metaphor 150, 153
visual schedule 116, 136-7, 161, 174
visual sensitivity 122, 131, 143, 170
visual sensory system 88, 97, 160, 174

Webb, James 28
working memory *43*, 43, 49, 51
WOW factor 119-21

Yates, Denise 101

Zones of Regulation 153

Printed in Great Britain
by Amazon